Mullaicharam Bhupathyraaj

Pharmaceutical Tablet Dosage Form- a Quick Review

Mullaicharam Bhupathyraaj

Pharmaceutical Tablet Dosage Form- a Quick Review

A Quick Review for Medical And Life Science Students

Noor Publishing

Imprint

Any brand names and product names mentioned in this book are subject to trademark, brand or patent protection and are trademarks or registered trademarks of their respective holders. The use of brand names, product names, common names, trade names, product descriptions etc. even without a particular marking in this work is in no way to be construed to mean that such names may be regarded as unrestricted in respect of trademark and brand protection legislation and could thus be used by anyone.

Cover image: www.ingimage.com

Publisher:
Noor Publishing
is a trademark of
Dodo Books Indian Ocean Ltd., member of the OmniScriptum S.R.L Publishing group
str. A.Russo 15, of. 61, Chisinau-2068, Republic of Moldova Europe
Printed at: see last page
ISBN: 978-620-3-86021-4

PHARMACEUTICAL TABLET DOSAGE FORM- A Quick Review:

Author:

Prof. MULLAICHARAM BHUPATHYRAAJ, Ph.D,

Professor of Pharmaceutics,

College of Pharmacy,

National University of Science and Technology,

P.O.Box 620: Postal code: 130: Azaiba,

Muscat, Sultanate of Oman.

2021

Table of Contents

		form	
		• Advantages and Disadvantages	
		• Methos of Preparation of Tablet Dosage forms	
		• Problems in Tableting	
5	Pharmaceutical Tablet Coating Technologies	• Tablet Coating concepts • History of coating, • Supercell Coating • Magnetically Assisted Impaction Coating	• 88-105
6	Evaluation of Pharmaceutical Tablets	• Description of quality control test • Weight variation test • Tablet Hardness test • Tablet Friability Test • Tablet Disintegration test • Tablet Dissolution test • Tablet Thickness test	• 106-118
7	Model Questions	• All chapters	• 119-136

Chapter-1

Introduction to Pharmaceutical Dosage Forms

Objectives

- After reading first part of this chapter, the student will be able to:

1. Define the dosage form design.

2. Describe the required features to ensure product quality.

3. Differentiate the various types of dosage forms based on route of administration.

4. Discuss the factors to be considered before formulated into dosage form

Principal objective of dosage form design

The principal objective of dosage form design is to achieve a predictable therapeutic response to a drug included in a formulation which is capable of large scale manufacture with reproducible product quality.

How to ensure quality of product?

- To ensure product quality, numerous features are required —

- ❖ chemical and physical stability,

- ❖ with suitable preservation against microbial contamination if appropriate,

- ❖ uniformity of dose of drug,

- ❖ acceptability to users including both prescriber and patient,

- ❖ as well as suitable packaging and labeling.

- Ideally, dosage forms should also be <u>independent of patient to patient variation</u> although in practice this feature remains <u>difficult to achieve.</u>

- Future developments in dosage form design may well attempt to accommodate to some extent this requirement.

- ❖ In recent years increasing attention has therefore been directed towards <u>eliminating variation in bioavailability characteristics</u>, particularly for <u>chemically equivalent</u>

3

products since it is recognized that formulation factors can influence their therapeutic performance.

A) Bioavailability

- Bioavailability refers to the extent and rate at which the active moiety (drug or metabolite) enters systemic circulation, thereby accessing the site of action.

B) Chemically equivalent products

- Chemical equivalence indicates that drug products contain the same active compound in the same amount and meet current official standards; however, inactive ingredients in drug products may differ.

- To optimize the bioavailability of drug substances it is often necessary to carefully select the most appropriate chemical derivative of the drug, for example to obtain a specific solubility requirement, as well as its particle size and physical form,

❖ **To combine it with appropriate additives and**

❖ **Manufacturing aids that will not significantly alter the properties of the drug,** (A manufacturing aid helps to run the equipment and is never incorporated into the product. Examples include lubricants, coolants, and refrigerants)

❖ **To select the most appropriate administration route(s) and dosage form(s) and to consider aspects of manufacturing processes and suitable packaging.**

- To optimize the bioavailability of drug substances

- it is often necessary to carefully select the most appropriate chemical derivative of the drug, for example to obtain a specific solubility requirement,

- Dosage forms can be designed for administration by all possible delivery routes to maximize therapeutic response.

- Preparations can be taken orally or injected, as well as being applied to the skin or inhaled, and Table 1 lists the range of dosage forms which can be used to deliver drugs by the various administration routes.

- However, it is necessary to <u>relate the drug substance and the disease state before the correct combination of drug and dosage form can be made</u> since each disease or illness will require a specific type of drug therapy.

- It is therefore apparent that before a drug substance can be successfully formulated into dosage form many factors must be considered. These can be broadly grouped into three categories:

- ❖   1. **Biopharmaceutical considerations,** including factors affecting the absorption of the drug substance from different administration routes,

- ❖   2. **Drug factors**, such as the physical and chemical properties of the drug substance, and

- ❖   3.**Therapeutic considerations** including consideration of the disease to be treated and factors

How can we achieve the principal objective of dosage form design?

- <u>Appropriate and efficacious dosage forms be prepared only when all these factors considered</u> and related to each other. <u>This is the underlying principle of dosage form design.</u>

- <u>**BIOPHARMACEUTICAL CONSIDERATIONS IN DOSAGE FORM DESIGN**</u>

- Biopharmaceutics can be regarded as **the study of the relationship between the physical, chemical and biological sciences applied to drugs, dosage forms and drug action**.

- In general, a <u>drug substance must be in solution</u> form before it can be absorbed via absorbing membranes of the skin, gastrointestinal tract and lungs into body fluids.

- Drugs penetrate these membranes in two general ways — <u>by passive diffusion and by specialized transport mechanisms.</u>

- Dosage forms can be designed for administration by all possible delivery routes to <u>maximize therapeutic response.</u>

- Preparations can be taken orally or injected, as well as being applied to the skin or inhaled, and Table 1.1 lists the range of dosage forms which can be used to deliver drugs by the various administration routes.

Table 1.1 Range of dosage forms available for different administration routes

Administration route	Dosage forms
Oral	Solutions, syrups, elixirs, suspensions, emulsions, gels, powders, granules, capsules, tablets
Rectal	Suppositories, ointments, creams, powders, solutions
Topical	Ointments, creams, pastes, lotions, gels, solutions, topical aerosols
Parenteral	Injections (solution, suspension, emulsion forms), implants, irrigation and dialysis solutions
Lungs	Aerosols (solution, suspension, emulsion, powder forms), inhalations, sprays, gases
Nasal	Solutions, inhalations
Eye	Solutions, ointments
Ear	Solutions, suspensions, ointments

• However, it is necessary to <u>relate the drug substance and the disease state before the correct combination of drug and dosage form can be made</u> since each disease or illness will require a specific type of drug therapy.

• It is therefore apparent that before a drug substance can be successfully formulated into dosage form many factors must be considered. These can be broadly grouped into three categories:

• 1. **Biopharmaceutical considerations**, including factors affecting the absorption of the drug substance from different administration routes,

• 2. **Drug factors**, such as the physical and chemical properties of the drug substance, and

• 3. **Therapeutic considerations** including consideration of the disease to be treated and factors.

- **How can we achieve the principal objective of dosage form design?**

- Appropriate and efficacious dosage forms be prepared only when all these factors considered and related to each other. This is the underlying principle of dosage form design.

- <u>BIOPHARMACEUTICAL CONSIDERATIONS IN DOSAGE FORM DESIGN</u>

- Biopharmaceutics can be regarded as **<u>the study of the relationship between the physical, chemical and biological sciences applied to drugs, dosage forms and drug action</u>**.

- In general, a <u>drug substance must be in solution</u> form before it can be absorbed via absorbing membranes of the skin, gastrointestinal tract and lungs into body fluids.

- Drugs penetrate these membranes in two general ways — <u>by passive diffusion and by specialized transport mechanisms.</u>

- **A) Passive diffusion**

- Passive transport is a movement of biochemical and other atomic or molecular substances across cell membranes. Unlike active transport, it does not require an input of chemical energy, being driven by the growth of entropy of the system.

- **B) Specialized transport mechanisms**

- In contrast to the passive transfer of drugs and other substances across a biologic membrane with the use of carrier.

- Once absorbed, the drug can exert a therapeutic effect yet <u>the site of action is often remote from the site of administration</u> and has to be transported in body fluids (see Fig. 1.1).

Schematic diagram illustrating pathways a drug may take following administration of a dosage form by different routes

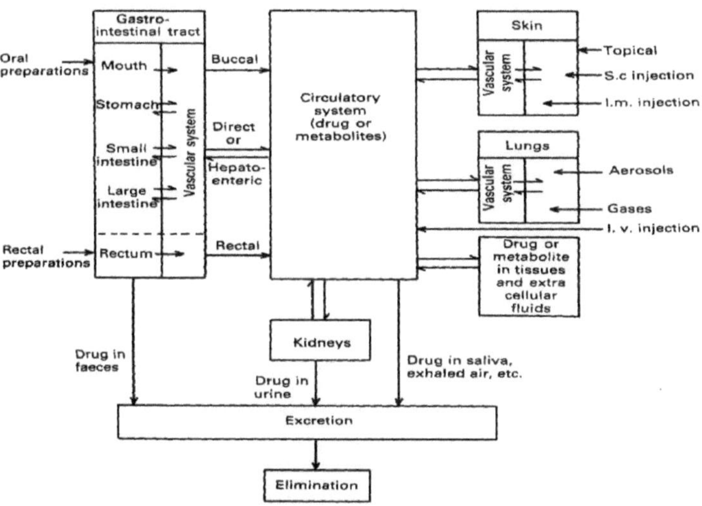

Fig. 1.1 Schematic diagram illustrating pathways a drug may take following administration of a dosage form by different routes

- **<u>Drug factors in dosage form design</u>**

- Each type of dosage form requires careful study of the physical and chemical properties of drug substances to achieve a stable, efficacious product.

- These properties such as

– dissolution,

– crystal size and polymorphic form,

– solid state stability and

– drug additive interaction, can have profound effects on the physiological availability and physical and chemical stability of the drug.

- By combining such data with those from pharmacological and biochemical studies, the most suitable drug form and additives can be selected for the formulation of chosen dosage forms

- Whilst, comprehensive property evaluation will not be required for all types of formulations those properties which are recognized as important in dosage form design and processing are listed in Table 1.3.

Table 1.3 Physical and chemical properties of drug substances important in dosage form design and potential stresses with range of manufacturing procedures used in processing

Properties	Processing stresses	Manufacturing procedures
Organoleptic	Temperature	Crystallization
Particle size, surface area	Pressure	Precipitation
	Mechanical	Filtration
Solubility	Radiation	Emulsification
Dissolution	Exposure to liquids	Milling
Partition coefficient	Exposure to gases and liquid vapours	Mixing
Ionization constant		Drying
Crystal properties, polymorphism		Granulation
		Compression
Stability		Autoclaving
(Other properties)		Handling
		Storage
		Transport

- Modern medicines require that pharmaceutical dosage forms are acceptable to the patient.

- Unfortunately many drug substances in use today are unpalatable and unattractive in their natural state and dosage forms, particularly oral preparations, containing such drugs may require the addition of approved flavors, perfumes and/or colors.

- **Particle size and surface area**

Particle size reduction results in an increase in the specific surface (i.e. surface area per unit weight) of powders.

- Drug dissolution rate, absorption rate, dosage form content uniformity and stability are all dependent to varying degrees on particle size, size distribution and interactions of solid surfaces.

- In many cases for <u>both drugs and additives particle size reduction is required to achieve the desired physicochemical characteristics.</u>

- **Solubility**

All drugs, whatever route they are administered by, must exhibit at least limited aqueous solubility for therapeutic efficiency.

- Thus relatively <u>insoluble compounds can exhibit erratic or incomplete absorption,</u> and it might be appropriate to use more soluble salt or ester derivatives.

- Alternatively, micronizing, complexation or solid dispersion techniques might be employed.

- Solubility can also be important in the absorption of drugs already in solution in liquid dosage forms since precipitation in the gastrointestinal tract can occur and bioavailability modified. Drug dissolution is slow due to its physicochemical properties or formulation factors, then dissolution may be the <u>rate-limiting step in absorption</u> and influence drug bioavailability.

- The dissolution of a drug is described by the general <u>Noyes—Whitney equation</u>:

$dm/dt = kA\ (C_s - C)$

where dm/dt is the dissolution rate,

– k is the dissolution rate constant,

– A is the surface area of dissolving solid,

– C_s is the concentration of drug in the saturated diffusing layer and

– C is the concentration of drug in the dissolution medium at time t.

- **Dissolution**

As mentioned above, for a drug to be absorbed it must <u>first be dissolved in *the* fluid at the site of absorption</u>.

- For example, an <u>orally administered</u> drug in tablet form is not absorbed until drug particles are dissolved or solubilized by the <u>fluids at some point along the gastrointestinal tract, depending on the pH-solubility profile of the drug substance</u>.

- Dissolution describes the **process** by which the drug particles dissolve.

- The equation reveals that <u>dissolution rate</u> can be raised by increasing the surface area (reducing particle size) of the drug,

- by increasing the solubility of the drug in the diffusing layer and

- by increasing k which incorporates the drug diffusion coefficient and diffusion layer thickness.

- Dissolution rate data when combined with <u>solubility, partition coefficient and *pKa*</u> results provide an insight to the formulator into the potential <u>*in vivo* absorption characteristics of a drug</u>.

- However, *in vitro* tests **only have significance** <u>if they can be related to *in vivo* results</u>.

- Once such a relationship has been established, <u>*in vitro* dissolution tests can be used as a quality control test</u>.

- **Partition coefficient and pKa** for relatively <u>insoluble compounds the dissolution rate is often the rate- determining step in the overall absorption process</u>.

- Alternatively, for <u>soluble compounds the rate of permeation across biological membranes is the rate-determining step</u>.

- Whilst <u>dissolution rate can be changed by</u>

  – **modifying the physicochemical properties of the drug and / or by**

  – **altering the formulation composition,**

- the permeation rate is dependent upon

  – the size,

–   relative aqueous and lipid solubility and

–   ionic charge of drug molecules,

–   Factors which can be altered through molecular modifications.

•   The absorbing membrane acts as a lipophilic barrier to the passage of drugs which is related to the lipophilic nature of the drug molecule.

•   <u>The partition coefficient, for example between oil and water, is a measure of lipophilic character.</u>

•   The majority of drugs are weak acids or bases and depending on the pH exist in an ionized or unionized form.

•   The factors therefore that <u>influence the absorption of weak acids and bases are</u>

–   The pH at the site of absorption

–   The lipid solubility of the unionized species.

•   **Crystal properties; polymorphism**

•   The different polymorphs vary in physical properties such as

–   solubility,

–   dissolution,

–   solid state stability

–   processing behavior in terms of powder flow and compaction during tableting.

•   Polymorphic transitions can also occur during <u>milling, granulating, drying and compressing operations</u>

•   Granulation can result in solvate formation or, during drying a solvated or hydrated molecule may be lost to form an anhydrous material.

•   Consequently, the formulator must be aware of these <u>potential transformations which can result in undesirable modified product performance, even though routine chemical analyses may not reveal any changes.</u>

- Reversion from metastable forms, if used, to the stable form may also occur during the lifetime of the product.

- **In suspensions,** this may be accompanied by <u>changes in the consistency</u> of the preparation which <u>affects its shelf life and stability</u>.

- Such changes can often be <u>prevented by additives, such as hydrocolloids and surface-active agents</u> which appear to poison the crystal lattice

Stability

- In general drug substances decompose as a result of the effects of heat, oxygen, light and moisture.

- For example, esters such as aspirin and procaine are susceptible to solvolytic breakdown, whilst oxidative decomposition occurs for substances such as ascorbic acid.

- Drugs can be classified according to their sensitivity to breakdown:

1. Stable at all conditions (e.g. kaolin),
2.stable if handled correctly (e.g. aspirin),
3. Moderately unstable even with special handling (e.g. vitamins),
4 very unstable (e.g. certain antibiotics in solution form).

- **Other drug properties**

- Other characteristics such as hygroscopicity, flowability and compressibility are particularly valuable when preparing solid dosage forms where the drugs constitute a large percentage of the formulation.

- **THERAPEUTIC CONSIDERATIONS IN DOSAGE FORM DESIGN**

- The nature of the disease or illness against which the drug is intended is an important factor when selecting the range of dosage forms to be prepared.

- Factors such as

- the need for systemic or local therapy,

- duration of action required and

- whether the drug will be used in emergency situations, need to be considered.

•	In the vast majority of cases a single drug substance is prepared into a number of dosage forms to satisfy both the particular preferences of the patient or physician and the specific needs of a certain situation.

•	For example many asthmatic patients use inhalation aerosols from which the drug is rapidly absorbed into the systematic circulation following deep inhalation.

•	In the vast majority of cases a single drug substance is prepared into a number of dosage forms to satisfy both the particular preferences of the patient or physician and the specific needs of a certain situation.

•	For example many asthmatic patients use inhalation aerosols from which the drug is rapidly absorbed into the systematic circulation following deep inhalation.

Pharmaceutical dosage forms   for systemic administration

•	Generations of dosage forms

–	1st gen. – conventional (unmodified) release of API

–	2nd gen. – controlled release of API (CR)

–	3rd gen. – targeted distribution drug delivery systems

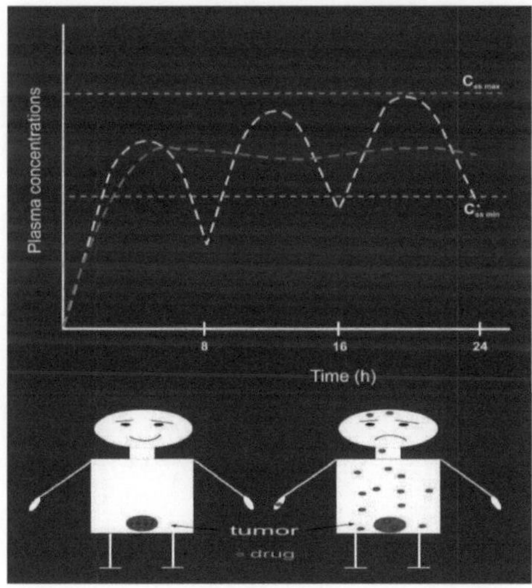

– **1st generation. – conventional (unmodified) release of API**

> ➢ Eg. Tablets, capsules.
> ➢ First order release and drug release at site of administration
> ➢ More side effects and less beneficial effects
> ➢ More frequency of administration and more dose required.

– **2nd generation. – controlled release of API (CR)**

> ➢ Eg. Transdermal, Matrix tablets and microencapsules.
> ➢ Zero order release and drug release at site of administration
> ➢ Less side effects and More beneficial effects
> ➢ Less frequency of administration and Less dose required

– **3rd generation. – targeted distribution drug delivery systems**

> ➢ Eg. Drug Nano particles, Liposomes, Niosomes.
> ➢ Zero order release and drug release at site of action
> ➢ Very Less side effects and More beneficial effects
> ➢ Very Less frequency of administration and Very Less dose required

- **Summary**

- The formulation and associated preparation of dosage forms demands careful examination, analysis and evaluation of wide ranging information by pharmaceutical scientists to achieve the objective of creating high quality and efficacious dosage forms.

References:

1. Allen, LV, Nicholas G, Ansel HC. Ansel's Pharmaceutical Dosage Forms and Drug Delivery Systems (9th ed.), Lippincott Williams & Wilkins, 2011(Latest edition).

2. Sinko PJ. Martin's Physical Pharmacy and Pharmaceutical Sciences (6th ed.), Lippincott Williams & Wilkins; 2010(Latest edition)

3. Aulton, M.E. Pharmaceutics: The Science of dosage form design, (2nd ed.), Churchill Livingstone, (Latest edition).

Chapter: 2

Preformulation Studies

Objectives

- After reading first part of this chapter, the student will be able to:

1. Define the Preformulation concepts.

2. Describe the required features of preformulation studied in solid dosage forms.

3. Describe the required features of preformulation studied in liquid dosage forms.

4. Describe the required features of preformulation studied in topical and inhalation dosage forms

Definition

Preformulation involves the application of biopharmaceutical principles to the physicochemical parameters of drug substance are characterized with the goal of designing optimum drug delivery system.

Preformulation commences when newly synthesized drug shows sufficient pharmacologic promise in animal model to warrant evaluate in man.

Biopharmaceutics:

The study of physical and chemical properties of drugs and their proper dosage form as related to the onset, duration and intensity of drug action.

The acidic or basic nature of the molecule can be predicted from the functional groups in its structure.

This will indicate suitable solvents to ensure solution of either the ionized or undissociated species.

INTRODUCTION

It is axiomatic that the physicochemical properties of candidate drugs can influence their subsequent development. The results of characterization studies carried out will influence their product design. However, in the interest of only doing necessary work, any detailed studies should only be carried out after the candidate drug has successfully overcome the safety and clinical trials performed in early development as many will fail at this stage. Since pharmaceuticals are formulated in a variety of dosage forms, the studies that should be undertaken include those of solid and solution state. In terms of solid-state evaluation, material science has assumed great importance and this is especially true for compounds to be delivered via the inhalation route. If the solid-state characteristics of the candidate drugs are less than desirable from a formulation perspective, then crystal engineering techniques can sometimes be employed to give them more amenable properties.

Variability of the drug candidate and excipients is the major cause of challenges in the formulation development of new compounds, and so methods for their characterization need to be available. While there are many traditional approaches to dosage form design, newer approaches based on expert systems that require knowledge of the physicochemical properties are being employed to speed up development.

SOLID DOSAGE FORMS

Since tablets and capsules account for approximately 70% of pharmaceutical preparations, an investigation into the solid-state properties of candidate drugs is an important task to be undertaken during preformulation. Generally speaking, when dealing with high strength solid dosage forms, this formulation will be more susceptible to any drug substance variability. However, other studies are also important since, for example, the same chemical compound can have different crystal structures (polymorphs), external shapes (habits), and hence different flow and compression properties.

<u>Impurities</u>

Since unwanted impurities, for example, intermediates, degradation products, and products from side reactions may have deleterious pharmacological and toxicological activities, they must be removed from the final product. The identification of impurities is thus a crucial activity in drug substance PR&D. Indeed, it is a regulatory requirement that the level of impurities in the drug substance be controlled. In addition to regulatory requirements, the incorporation of impurities in the crystal lattice can lead to crystal defects, which in turn can lead to differences in, for example, mechanical properties, dissolution behavior, and stability, which may be the basis of batch-to-batch variation. One of the main objectives of crystallization is therefore to purge the compound of these impurities to make it fit for use as the active pharmaceutical ingredient in a medicine.

ICH classifies impurities into the following categories: organic impurities (process and drug related), inorganic impurities, and residual solvents. Organic impurities include, starting materials, by-products, intermediates, degradation products as well as reagents, ligands, and catalysts. Inorganic impurities can often result from the manufacturing process, and examples of these are reagents, ligands and catalysts, heavy metals, inorganic salts, and other process-related materials such as filtration aids and charcoal. Solvents are controlled though ICH guideline Q3C. In addition to these obvious impurities, polymorphs as well as enantiomeric impurities need to be considered.

Impurities can have effects on the size, shape, and polymorphic form of compounds, such that, as the synthetic chemists experiment with different synthetic routes to the drug substance, different impurities generated can alter the physical properties of the crystals generated.

Impurities may also affect the polymorph that crystallizes from solution. The most important learning point of these studies is that the presence of impurities can affect the results of polymorph screens, since impurities can stabilize metastable forms and give a false sense of security that you are dealing with the stable form. Therefore, the use of pure material for polymorph screens is recommended, and the screen should be reconducted when route changes are made—especially if the impurity profile changes.

It should also remembered that formulations also contain excipients that have their own crystal properties, which can be altered by the incorporation of impurities with the result that batch-to-batch variation can be experienced..

<u>Polymorphism Issues</u>

Because polymorphism can have an effect on so many aspects of drug development, it is important to fix the polymorph (usually the stable form) as early as possible in the development cycle and probably before campaign.

While it is hoped that the issue polymorphism is resolved during prenomination and early development, it can remain a concern when the synthesis of the drug is scaled up into a larger reactor or transferred to another production site. In extreme cases and despite intensive research, work may have only produced a metastable form and the first production batch produces the stable form.

The following scheme should be followed in the production of Candidate Drugs

 1. Selection of the solvent system

2. Characterization of the polymorphic forms

3. Optimization of process times, temperature, solvent compositions, etc.

4. Examination of the chemical stability of the drug during processing

5. Manipulation of the polymorphic form, if necessary

While examples of disappearing polymorphs exist, perhaps more common is the crystallization of mixtures of polymorphs. Many analytical techniques have been used to quantitate mixtures of polymorphs. Moreover, while the production of the forms may be straightforward, production of homogeneously mixed samples for calibration purposes may not be so. To overcome this problem, a slurry technique was employed, which satisfied the NDA requirements, to determine the amount of one form in the other. The criteria employed are as follows:

1. A polymorphic transformation did not occur during preparation or analysis.

2. A limit of detection of 5% (w/w) of the dihydrate in monohydrate.

3. Ease of sample preparation, data acquisition, and analysis.

4. Ease of transfer to a quality control (QC) environment.

Calibration samples were limited to a working range of 1% to 15% w/w, and to prepare the mixes, samples of each form were slurried in acetone to produce a homogeneous mixture of the two.

With respect to solid dosage forms, there have been a few reports on how processing affects the polymorphic behavior of compounds.

Solvate formation may have some advantages. The desolvated dioxane solvate of nimesulide had better tableting properties than the known polymorphs of the compound, which appears to represent a viable method of improving the compression properties of drug substances.

Polymorphism is not only an issue with the compound under investigation, that is, excipients also show variability in this respect. It is well known that polymorphism is a function of temperature and pressure, thus under the compressive forces that compounds experience under tableting conditions phase transformations may be possible.

SOLUTION FORMULATIONS

Development of a solution formulation requires a number of key pieces of preformulation information. Of these, solubility (and any pH dependence) and stability are probably the most important.

Solubility Considerations

One of the main problems associated with developing a parenteral or any other solution formulation of a compound is its aqueous solubility. For a poorly soluble drug candidate, there are several strategies for enhancing its solubility. These include pH manipulation, cosolvents, surfactants, emulsion formation, and complexing agents; combinations of these methods can also be used. More sophisticated delivery systems, for example, liposomes, can also be considered.

pH Manipulation

Since many compounds are weak acids or bases, their solubility will be function of pH. The pH-solubility curve for sibenadit HCl salt with pKas at 6.58 and 8.16. When the acid-base titration method was used, the solubility curve showed a minimum pH between 6 and 8. Below this pH region, the solubility increased as the pKa was passed to reach a maximum between pH 2 and 4 and then decreased because of the common ion effect. As the second pKa was passed in the alkaline region, the solubility again increased. However, when the solubility experiments were performed in 0.2 M citrate phosphate buffer, the solubility of the compound decreased, and this illustrates the effect that ionic strength can have on drug solubility. Clearly, the region between pH 2 and 5 represents the best area to achieve the highest solubility. However, caution should be exercised if the solution needs to be buffered, since this can decrease the solubility, as in this case. It was found that a buffered formulation of a compound did not precipitate on dilution and did not cause phlebitis. In contrast, the unbuffered drug formulation showed the opposite effects. These results reinforce the importance of buffering parenteral formulations instead of simply adjusting the pH.

Cosolvents

The use of cosolvents has been utilized quite effectively for some poorly soluble drug substances. It is probable that the mechanism of enhanced solubility is the result of the polarity of the cosolvent mixture being closer to the drug than in water. It was found that the aprotic cosolvents gave a much higher degree of solubility than the amphiprotic cosolvents. This means that if a cosolvent can donate a hydrogen bond, it may be an important factor in determining whether it is a good cosolvent.

While cosolvents can increase the solubility of compounds, on occasion, they can have a detrimental effect on their stability. For example, a parenteral formulation of the novel antitumor agent carzelsin (U80,244) using a PEG 400/absolute ethanol/polysorbate 80 PET) formulation in the ratio 6:3:1 v/v/v has been reported . While this formulation effectively increased the solubility of the compound, this work showed that interbatch variation of PEG 400 could affect the stability of the drug because of pH effects.

One point that is often overlooked when considering cosolvents is their influence on buffers or salts. Since these are conjugate acid-base systems, it is not surprising that introducing solvents into the solution can result in a shift in the pKa of the buffer or salt. These effects are important in formulation terms, since many injectable formulations that contain cosolvents also contain a buffer to control the pH .

Emulsion Formulations

Oil-in-water (o/w) emulsions have been successfully employed to deliver drugs with poor water solubility. In preformulation terms, the solubility of the compound in the oil phase (often soybean oil) is the main consideration while using this approach. However, the particle size of the emulsion and its stability (physical and chemical) also need to be assessed. Ideally, the particle size of the emulsion droplets should be in the colloidal range to avoid problems with phlebitis. To achieve this size, a microfluidizer should be used, since other techniques may produce droplets of a larger size. Emulsions are prepared by homogenizing the oil in water in the presence of emulsifiers, for example, phospholipids, which stabilize the emulsion via a surface charge and also a mechanical barrier. Intravenous emulsions can be sterilized by autoclaving, which gives a high level of assurance of sterility.

However, careless aseptic techniques can compromise the patient. In this situation, the inclusion of antimicrobial additives could be considered.

The particle size and zeta potential of emulsions can be measured using instruments that combine PCS and surface charge measurements. It have compared a light obscuration (LO) and laser diffraction to examine the stability of parenteral nutrition mixtures–based intravenous emulsions. From this study, they concluded that LO was a better technique for detecting globules greater than 5 mm in diameter. They recommended two key measurements, that is, the mean droplet size and the large droplet size, since without these it is impossible to guarantee the safety of the emulsion (large droplets can cause thrombophlebitis)

Stability Considerations

The second major consideration with respect to solution formulations is stability. The stability of pharmaceuticals, from a regulatory point of view, is usually determined by forced degradation studies. These studies provide data on the identity of degradants, degradation pathways, and the fundamental stability of the molecule. Guidance for the industry on how to conduct stability testing of new drug substances and products is given in the ICH guideline

SUSPENSIONS

If the drug substance is not soluble, then the compound may be administered as a suspension. This might be the formulation approach used for oral administration of drugs to animals for safety studies, for early-phase clinical studies in humans, or for the intended commercial dosage form, for example, ophthalmic, nasal, oral, etc. Data considered to be important for suspensions at the preformulation stage include solubility, particle size, and propensity for crystal growth and chemical stability. Furthermore, during development, it will be important to have knowledge of the viscosity of the vehicle to obtain information with respect to settling of the suspended particles, syringibility, and physical stability. In a report on the preformulation information required for suspensions, It has been investigated the relationship between the critical volume fraction as a function of pH. They noted that "it is usually desirable to maximize the volume fraction of solids to minimize the volume of the dose."

It should be obvious that for a successful suspension, insolubility of the candidate drug is required. While for large hydrophobic drugs like steroids, this may not be a problem, weak acids or bases may show appreciable solubility. In this instance, reducing the solubility by salt formation is a relatively common way to achieve this end. For example, a calcium salt of a weak acid may be sufficiently insoluble for a suspension formulation. However, difficulties may arise because of hydrate formation, for example, with concomitant crystal growth. It was found that metronidazole formed a monohydrate on suspension in water.This conversion can be prevented by using Avicel RC-591 as a suspending agent.

The crystal habit may also affect the physical stability of the formulation.

If the suspension is for parenteral administration, it will need to be sterilized. However, terminal heat sterilization can affect both its chemical and physical stabilities, the latter usually observed as crystal growth or aggregation of the particles .Another measure of suspension stability is the zeta potential, which is a measure of the surface charge. However, various studies have shown that it is only useful in some cases.

As noted above, the particle size of suspensions is another important parameter in suspension formulations. The particle size distribution can be measured using a variety of techniques including laser diffraction. A point to note in laser diffraction is the careful selection of the suspending agent.

The particle size of the suspensions was measured as a function of time, and surprisingly, Tween 80, which is widely used in this respect, was found to be unsuitable for the hydrophobic drug under investigation. Other surfactants also gave poor particle size data, for example, Tween 20, Cetomacrogol 1000, Pluronic F88, and sodium lauryl sulfate. This arose from aggregation of the particles, and additionally, these suspensions showed slower drug dissolution into water. Span 20 and Pluronic L62 showed the best results, and the authors cautioned the use of a standard surface active agent in preclinical studies.

Usually, suspensions are flocculated so that the particles form large aggregates that are easy to disperse—normally, this is achieved using potassium or sodium chloride. However, for controlled flocculation suspensions, sonication may be required to determine the size of the primary particles.

Although high performance liquid chromatography (HPLC) is the preferred technique for assessing the stability of formulations, spectrophotometry can also be used.

TOPICAL/TRANSDERMAL FORMULATIONS

Preformulation aspects of transdermal drug delivery offers several potential advantages compared with the oral route such as avoidance of fluctuating blood levels, no first-pass metabolism, and no degradation attributable to stomach acid. However, the transdermal route is limited because of the very effective barrier function of the skin. Large, polar molecules do not penetrate the stratum corneum well. The physicochemical properties of candidate drugs that are important in transdermal drug include molecular weight and volume, aqueous solubility, melting point, and log P.

Clearly, these are intrinsic properties of the molecule and as such will determine whether or not the compounds will penetrate the skin. Furthermore, since many compounds are weak acids or bases, pH will have an influence on their permeation.

One way in which the transport of zwitterionic drugs though skin has been enhanced was to form a salt. The rank order of epidermal flux of the salts of phenylalanine across the epidermis was hydrobromide > hydrochloride > hydrofluoride > phenylalanine. Thus, like most other delivery routes, it is worth considering salt selection issues at the preformulation stage to optimize the delivery of the compound via the skin.

The formulation in which the candidate drug is applied to the skin is another important factor that can affect its bioavailability. In transdermal drug delivery, a number of vehicles may be used, such as creams, ointments, lotions, and gels. The solubility of the compound in the vehicle needs to be determined. Problems can arise from crystal growth if the system is supersaturated; for example, phenylbutazone creams were observed to have a gritty appearance attributable to crystal growth. Indeed, in matrix patches, crystals of estradiol hemihydrate or gestodene of up to 800 mm grew during three months of storage at room temperature. Needle-like crystals of the hydrate of betamethasone-17 valerate were found when creams were placed on storage.

Chemical and physical stability also needs to be considered. The dithranol showed a distinct instability in the paraffin base due to light, but was stable when protected from light. In terms of kinetics, it was found that the degradation in a topical cream and that in ethanol-water solutions were very similar in the pH range 2 to 6. This suggested that the degradation of this compound occurred in an aqueous phase or compartment that was undisturbed by the oily cream excipients. If the compound decomposes because of oxidation, then an antioxidant may have to be incorporated. In an attempt to reduce the photo degradation of a development compound, and compared the free acid of compound with a number of its salts, each of which they incorporated into a white soft paraffin base. Their results showed that after a one hour exposure in a SOL2 light-simulation cabinet, the disodium salt showed significant degradation.

The stability of 8-methoxypsoralen (8-MOP) in various ointments. They found that after 12 weeks of storage, the drug was stable in Unguentum Cordes and Cold Cream Naturel. However, the Unguentum Cordes emulsion began to crack after eight weeks. When formulated in a carbopol gel, 8-MOP was unstable. The physical structure of creams has been investigated by a variety of techniques, for example, DSC, TGA, microscopy, reflectance measure, rheology, Raman spectroscopy, and dielectric analysis (Peramal et al., 1997). Focusing on TGA and rheology, it was found that when aqueous BP creams were analyzed by TGA, there were two peaks in the derivative curve. It was concluded that these were attributable to the loss of free and lamellar water from the cream, and therefore TGA could be used as a quality-control tool. The lamellar structure of creams can also be confirmed using small-angle X-ray measurements. For example, the lamellar spacings of a sodium lauryl sulfate, cetostearyl alcohol and liquid paraffin cream were found to increase in size as the water content of the cream increased until, at greater than 60% water, the lamellar structure broke down. This was correlated with earlier work that showed that at this point, the release of hydrocortisone was increased.

It was reported the use of a laser diffraction method to measure the particle size of drugs dispersed in ointments. In this study, they stressed the fact that a very small particle size was required to ensure efficacy of the drug. In addition, the size of the particles was especially important if the ointment was for ophthalmic use where particles must be less than 25 mm. While the particle size of the suspended particles can be assessed microscopically, laser diffraction offers a more rapid analysis.

INHALATION DOSAGE FORMS

As noted by research, delivering drugs via the lung is not new since the absorption of nicotine by smoking of tobacco has been known for centuries, and before inhalation drug delivery devices, some asthma medications were administered in cigarettes. In addition, anesthetic gases are routinely administered by inhalation. For many years now, however, respiratory diseases such as asthma and chronic obstructive pulmonary disease (COPD) have been treated by inhaling the drug from a pressurized metered-dose inhaler (pMDI), DPI, or a nebulizer solution. Although pMDIs remain the most popular devices for the delivery of drugs to the lungs, DPIs have gained in popularity over the years.

Because of the large surface area available, drug delivery via the lung has a number of advantages over the oral route since the rate of absorption of small molecules from the lung is only bettered by the intravenous route, and thus the bioavailability is usually higher than that obtained from drug delivery by the oral route. However, drug deposition in the lung can be problematic and requires the drug to be reduced in size to between 2 and 6 mm for optimal effect. If the particle size is greater than 6 mm, the compound is deposited in the mouth and esophageal region, and there is no clinical effect apart from the part that is swallowed. Particles of size 2 mm, on the other hand, are deposited in the peripheral airways/alveoli

COMPATIBILITY

Compatibility studies are conducted to accelerate the development of formulations by allowing formulators to eliminate those excipients that cause API degradation. Factors that affect the compatibility between drugs and potential formulation aids include local pH and water content, which affect the chemical stability of the API. When conducting compatibility studies, there are four steps to be considered, which are as follows:

1. Sample preparation

2. Statistical design

3. Storage conditions

4. Method of analysis

Traditionally, a binary mixture of drug and the excipient being investigated is intimately mixed, the ratio of drug to excipient being often 1:1; however, other mixtures may also be investigated. These powder samples, one set of which is moistened, are then sealed into ampoules to prevent moisture loss. These are then stored at a suitable temperature and analyzed at various time points using HPLC, DSC, FTIR (Fourier transform infra-red), or TGA as appropriate.

Using DSC alone is not recommended since it can throw up false negatives and positives and should be used as guide only. Indeed, it has been have concluded that DSC experiments need to be supported by other techniques such as FTIR and HPLC. The use of microthermal analytical technologies such as localized thermomechanical analysis (L-TMA), localized differential thermal analysis (L-DTA), nanosampling, thermally assisted particle manipulation (TAPM), and photothermal microspectrometry (PTMS) . However, that these are quite specialized techniques not widely available in industry at this point in time. Alternatively, the drug in suspension with excipients may be investigated.

The original protocol for DSC compatibility testing was proposed by van Dooren (1983), who suggested the following scheme:

1. Run the drug candidate and excipients individually

2. Run mixtures of the drug candidate and excipients immediately after mixing

3. Run the drug candidate and excipients individually after three weeks at 558C

4. Run the drug candidate–excipient mix after three weeks at 558C

5. Run the single components and mixtures after three weeks at 558C only if the curves of the mixtures before and after storage at this temperature differ from each other. An excipient that is particularly desired may be investigated further by examining different weight ratios with the drug. This, it was claimed, would use a small amount of the candidate drug and also take into account factors such as mixing, granulation, and compression. Then only if the tablet is proven to be unstable, should retrospective examination of the incompatibility be undertaken

to identify the excipients that are incompatible. Indeed, according to this author, any formulations that do not contain lactose and magnesium stearate should be successful!

Other investigators may have different experiences and may not have access to a compaction simulator. It is also worth being aware of processing-induced incompatibilities such as that reported, who found that even after conventional compatibility testing, degradation of their compound in a trial formulation was observed. The incompatibility was traced to an unusual anhydrate-to-amorphous transition that occurred because of granulation. A new dry process was developed, and polarized light microscopy was used to confirm the presence of the crystalline anhydrate after formulation. Like other aspects of the work in the modern pharmaceutical industry, automation and high-throughput techniques are being employed to speed up the process.

At various time points, the mixtures were analyzed using fast gradient HPLC. Combined with the statistical experimental design factor interaction plots can be generated, and all this can be achieved using 0.1 mg of compound per data point.

3. MELTING POINT

- Capillary melting

- Hot stage microscopy (Hot stage in polarizable microscope)

- Differential scanning calorimetric thermal analysis (Exothermic / endothermic-recorded in chart)

A polymorph is a solid material with at least two different molecular arrangements each of which gives a distinct crystal species.

The lowest melting species is generally stable and other polymorphs are metastable and convert to the stable form.

There are also large differences in their physical properties so that they behave as distinct chemical entities.

Lowest melting species   More Stable

Highest melting species   Less Stable

Different physical properties for different polymorph of same drug.

So each polymorph is considered as separate chemical entities.

4. ASSAY DEVELOPMENT (Purity of drug in dosage forms)

(Quantitative Assay measures the amount of drug present in dosage forms)

Example: Turbidimetry, Disc plate method, Titrimetry.

Certain U.V techniques are worthy of discussion:

1. Solubility

2. Molecular weight

3. PKa

4. Assay (potency)

5. DRUG AND PRODUCT STABILITY

Drug degradation occurs by four main process

   (a) Hydrolysis – due to hydrogen

   (b) Oxidation – due to oxygen

   (c) Photolysis – due to Photons

   (d) Trace metal catalysis.

6 .MICROSCOPY

The microscope has two major applications in pharmaceutical preformulation:

(a) Basic crystallography, to determine crystal morphology (structure and habit), polymorphism and solvates

(b) Particle size analysis. (Microscope-eyepiece &stage micrometer)

7. POWDER FLOW PROPERTIES

Powder flow properties of primary importance to the formulator when handling a drug powder is an assessment of its flow properties

Bulk density - Weight of powder/bulk volume

Angle of repose $-\tan\theta =$ height / radius

8. COMPRESSION PROPERTIES

➢ Information on the compression properties of the pure drug is extremely useful.

➢ The tableted material should be plastic, i.e. capable of permanent deformation

➢ it should also exhibit a degree of brittleness (fragmentation).

➢ Accordingly if the drug dose is high and it behaves plastically, the chosen excipients should fragment, e.g. lactose, calcium phosphate.

➢ If the drug is brittle or elastic, the excipients should be plastic, e.g. microcrystalline cellulose, or plastic binders could be used in wet massing.

The compression properties

1. Elasticity –very little permanent changes during compression

2. Plasticity - permanent changes during compression

3. Fragmentabiity – more broken off

4. Punch filming propensity (sticking tendency) for small quantities of a new drug candidate can be established.

Conclusion

Preformulation is a learning phase about a drug

Preformulation studies have a significant part to play in anticipating formulation problems.

The main goal of preformulation studies is Innovative, stable, safe, cost- effective dosage forms capable of delivering the substance for its intended use.

REFERENCES

1. Pharmaceutical preformulation and formulation: A practical guide from candidate drug selection to commercial dosage form / edited by Mark Gibson. —2nd Ed, Volume 199, Page 188 – 247.

2. Allen, LV, Nicholas G, Ansel HC. Ansel's Pharmaceutical Dosage Forms and Drug Delivery Systems (9th ed.), Lippincott Williams & Wilkins, 2011(Latest edition).

3. Sinko PJ. Martin's Physical Pharmacy and Pharmaceutical Sciences (6th ed.), Lippincott Williams & Wilkins; 2010(Latest edition)

4. Aulton, M.E. Pharmaceutics: The Science of dosage form design, (2nd ed.), Churchill Livingstone, (Latest edition).

Chapter: 3

Granulation techniques and technologies:

Objectives

- ❑ Definition and concept
- ❑ Reasons for granulation
- ❑ Objective and Mechanism
- ❑ Methods for granulation process
- ➢ Direct compression
- ➢ Dry Compression
- ➢ Wet granulation

Granulation: Definition & concept

Granulation is a technique of particle enlargement by agglomeration in the production of tablets and capsules.

- Granulation is the process in which powder particles are made to adhere to form larger particles called granules.

- Powders/Granules intended for <u>compression</u> into <u>tablets</u> must possess <u>two essential properties</u> :

- <u>Flow property:</u> Flow property is required to produce tablets of a consistent weight and uniform strength

       Compressibility: <u>Compressibility</u> is required to form a <u>stable, intact compact mass</u> when pressure is applied.

These two objectives are obtained by granulation process. Granules so formed should possess acceptable flow property and compressibility

31

■   In the production of tablets or capsules, granules will be made as an intermediate product.

■   Granules may also be used as a dosage form.

■   Granulation will commence after mixing the necessary powdered ingredients so that a uniform distribution of each ingredient through the mix is achieved.

■   After granulation, the granules will be packed when used as a dosage form or they may be mixed with other excipients prior to tablet compression or capsule filling.

■   Granulation, a technique of particle enlargement by agglomeration, is one of the most significant unit operations in the production of pharmaceutical dosage forms, mostly tablets and capsules. During the granulation process, small fine or coarse particles are converted into large agglomerates called granules. Generally, granulation commences after initial dry mixing of the necessary powder ingredients along with the active pharmaceutical ingredient (API), so that a uniform distribution of each ingredient throughout the powder mixture is achieved. Although granules used in the pharmaceutical industry have particle size in the range of 0.2-4.0 mm, they are primarily produced as an intermediary with a size range of 0.2-0.5 mm to be either packed as a dosage form or be mixed with other excipients before tablet compaction or capsule filling.

■   Granules are produced to enhance the uniformity of the API in the final product, to increase the density of the blend so that it occupies less volume per unit weight for better storage and shipment, to facilitate metering or volumetric dispensing, to reduce dust during granulation process to reduce toxic exposure and process-related hazards, and to improve the appearance of the product. Consequently, the ideal characteristics of granules include spherical shape for improved flow, narrow particle size distribution for content uniformity and volumetric dispensing, sufficient fines to fill void spaces between granules for better compaction and compression characteristics, and adequate moisture and hardness to prevent breaking and dust formation during process.

■   Granulation is an exemplary of particle design and the properties of the particles acquired after granulation depend on particle size of the drug and excipients, the type, concentration, and volume of binder and/or solvents, granulation time, type of granulator, drying rate (temperature and time), etc. The primary methods by which the agglomerated granules are formed include solid bridges, sintering, chemical reaction, crystallization and deposition of colloidal particles. Besides, binding can also be accomplished through adhesive and cohesive forces by utilizing high viscous binders. The series of mechanisms by which granules are formed from the powder particles encompass wetting and nucleation, coalescence or growth, consolidation, and attrition or breakage.

- Blend of powders containing pharmaceutical excipients and API can be compressed into tablets either by direct compression or after making granules by agglomeration or granulation techniques. The granulation technique may be widely categorized in to two types, dry granulation and wet granulation, based on the type of method used to facilitate the agglomeration of powder particles. Dry granulation uses mechanical compression (slugs) or compaction (roller compaction) to facilitate the agglomeration of dry powder particles, while the wet granulation uses granulation liquid (binder/solvent) to facilitate the agglomeration by formation of wet mass by adhesion. Among these two techniques, wet granulation is the most widespread granulation technique used despite the fact that it involves multiple unit processes such as wet massing, drying and screening, which are complex, time consuming, and expensive requiring large space and multiple equipment.

- <u>Reasons for granulation</u>

1.*To prevent segregation of the constituents in the powder mix*
2.*To improve the flow properties of the mix*

- *3.To improve the compression characteristics of the mix*

4.*Other reasons*

Other reasons

1 .The granulation of toxic materials will reduce the hazard of the generation of toxic dust which may arise when handling powders.

- Suitable precautions must be taken to ensure that such dust is not a hazard during the granulation process.

2 .Materials which are slightly hygroscopic may adhere and form a cake if stored as a powder.

Granulation may reduce this hazard as the granules will be able to absorb some moisture and yet retain their flow ability because of their size.

◙   3. Granules, being denser than the parent powder mix, occupy less volume per unit weight.

■   They are therefore more convenient for storage or shipment.

<u>Objective and mechanism</u>

◙   The objective of the granulation process is to combine ingredients to produce a quality tablet.

◙   Granulation is process of collecting particles together bonds between then and these <u>bonds are formed by compression or by using a binding agent.</u>

◙   Particles-particles bonding mechanisms involved in adhesion and cohesion of particles.

◙   Several forces the can be act:

■   Valency,

■   Van der waals forces

■   Electrostatic forces

◙   <u>PARTICLE BONDING MECHANISMS</u>

◙   To form granules, bonds must be formed between powder particles so that they adhere and these bonds must be sufficiently strong to prevent breakdown of the granule to powder in subsequent handling operations.

◙   Rumpf (1962) distinguished five primary bonding mechanisms between particles:

◙   **1. Adhesion and cohesion forces in immobile liquid films,**

2. Interfacial forces in mobile liquid films,

3. Solid bridges,

4. Attractive forces between solid particles,

5. Interlocking bonds.

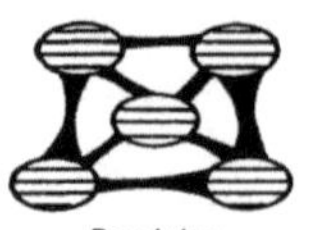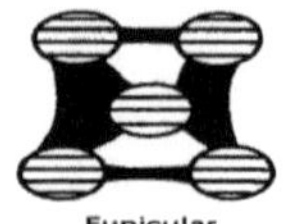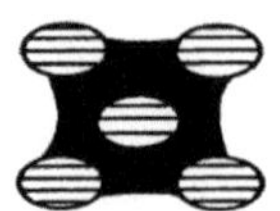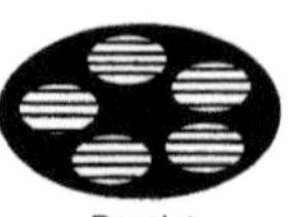

Fig. 37.2 Water distribution between particles

Interfacial forces in mobile liquid films

- Pendular

- Funicular

- Final Capillary

- <u>MECHANISMS OF GRANULE FORMATION</u>

1.**Nucleation**

2.**Transition**

3.**Ball growth**

- Coalescence

- Breakage

- Abrasion transfer

- Layering

- **<u>Nucleation</u>**

- Granulation starts with particle—particle contact and adhesion due to liquid bridges.

- A number of particles will join to form the pendular state.

- Further agitation densifies the pendular bodies to form the capillary state and these bodies act as nuclei for further granule growth.

- **<u>Transition</u>**

Nuclei can grow by two possible mechanisms:

- Either single particles can be added to the nuclei by pendular bridges or two or more nuclei may combine.

- The combined nuclei will be reshaped by the agitation of the bed.

This stage is characterized by the presence of a large number of small granules with a fairly wide size distribution

- **<u>Ball growth</u>**

- <u>Further granule growth produces large, spherical granules</u> and the mean particle size of the granulating system will increase with time.

- <u>If agitation is continued, granule coalescence will continue and produce an unusable, over massed system</u> although this is dependent upon the amount of liquid added and the properties of the material being granulated.

- *Coalescence*

- Two or more granules join to form a larger granule.

- *Breakage*

- Granules break into fragments which adhere to other granules forming a layer of material over the surviving granule.

- *Abrasion transfer*

- Agitation of the granule bed leads to attrition of material from granules.

- This abraded material adheres to other granules, increasing their size.

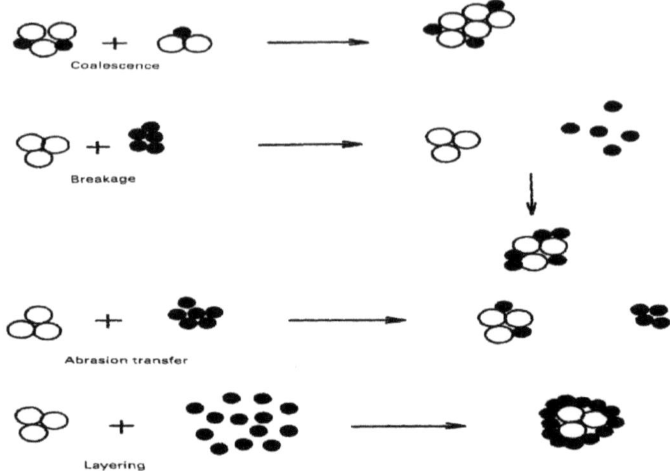

Fig. 37.3 Mechanisms of ball growth during granulation

◪ *Layering*

When <u>a second batch of powder mix is added to a bed of granules, the powder will adhere to the granules forming a layer</u> over the surface increasing the granule size

◪ <u>Methods of granulation</u>

1. *Dry granulation*

2. Wet granulation (or wet massing)

◪ Wet methods which utilize a liquid in the process and

Dry methods in which no liquid is used.

▪ In a suitable formulation a number of different excipients will be needed in addition to the drug.

▪ The common types used are diluents, to produce a unit dose weight of suitable size and

▪ disintegrating agents(**Disintegrants** are agents added to formulations to promote the breakup of the tablet into smaller fragments in an aqueous environment thereby increasing the available surface area and promoting a more rapid release of the drug substance.) which are added to disintegrate the granule in a liquid medium,

-     Adhesives in the form of a dry powder may also be added, particularly if dry granulation is employed.

-     These ingredients will be mixed before granulation.

- **<u>FILLERS</u>**

-     spray dried lactose,

-     microcrystals of alpha-monohydrate lactose,

-     sucrose-invert sugar-corn starch mixtures,

-     MCC, and

-     dicalcium phosphate

- **<u>Disintegrating agents</u>**

-     Direct compression starch,

-     Sodium carboxymethylstarch, etc.

- **<u>Lubricants</u>**

- mag.stearate

- talc

- **<u>Glidants-</u>**fumed silicon dioxide

- In simpler words, binders or adhesives are the substances that promotes cohesiveness. It is utilized for converting powder into granules through a process known as Granulation

- **Glidants. Glidants** are used to promote powder flow by reducing interparticle friction and cohesion.

- These are used in combination with **lubricants** as they have no ability to reduce die wall friction.

- *<u>Dry granulation</u>*

in the dry methods of granulation the powder particles are aggregated using high pressure.

- There are two main processes.

- Either a large tablet (known as a 'slug') is produced in a heavy duty tableting press (a process known as 'slugging') or

- Squeezed between two rollers to produce a sheet of material ('roller compaction').

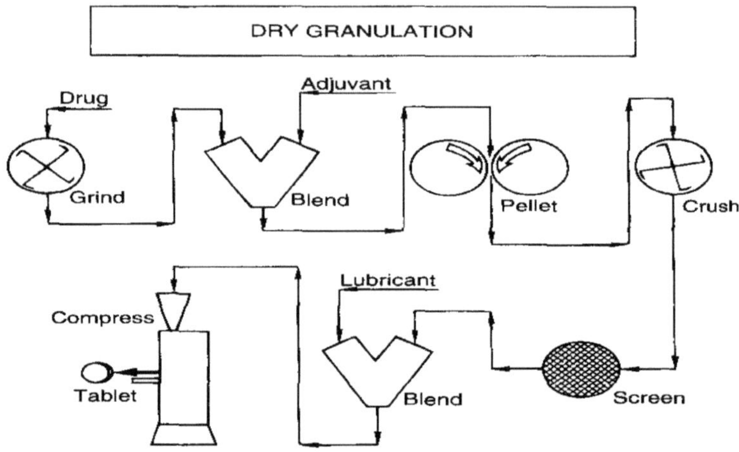

Tablet Press

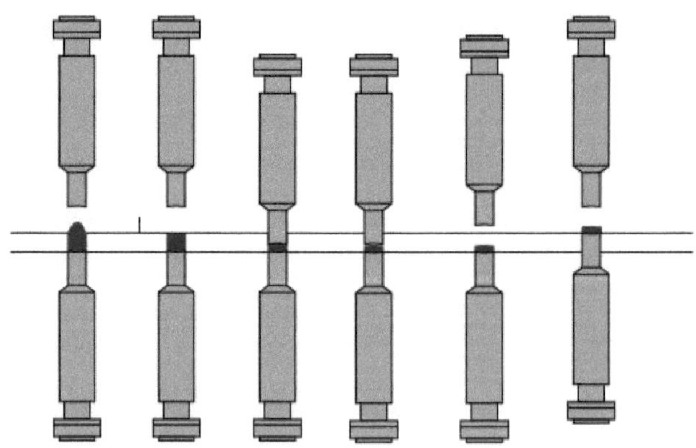

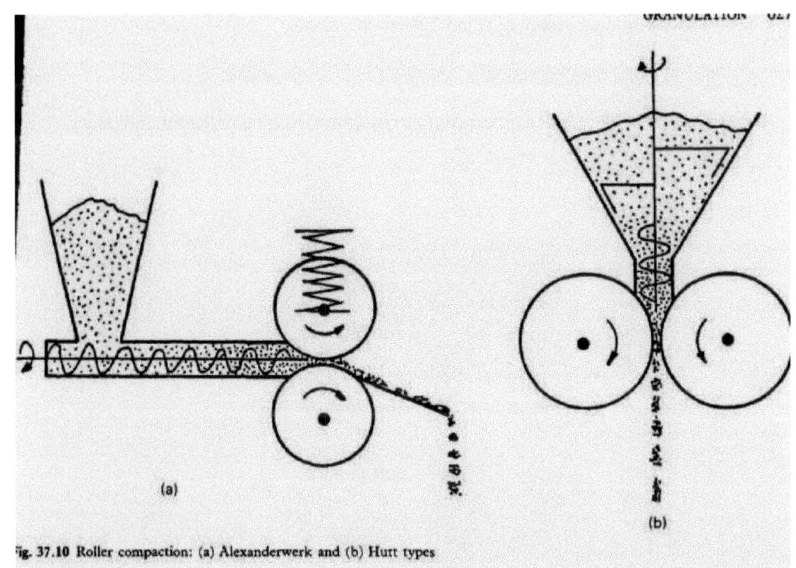

Fig. 37.10 Roller compaction: (a) Alexanderwerk and (b) Hutt types

Roller compactor

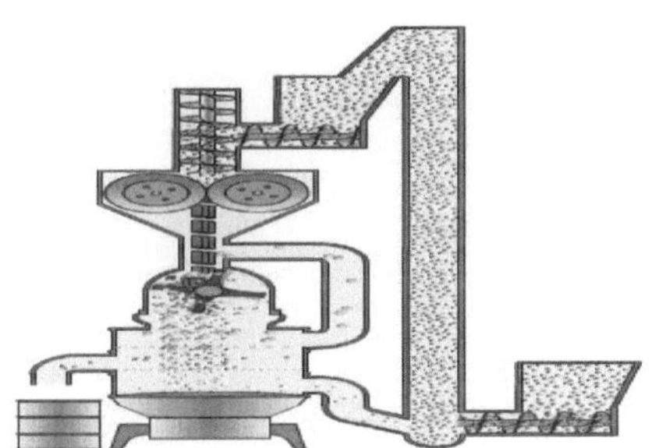

◘   <u>Slugging</u>

◘   After weighing and mixing the ingredients, powder mix. is slugged, or compressed into <u>large flat tablets or pellets about 1'' in dia.</u>

◘   Slugs are broken up

◘   by hand or

◘   by a mill and

40

◘   Passed through screen of desired mesh for sizing.

Lubricant added in usual manner and tablets prepared by compression.

◘   Aspirin, which is hydrolyzed on exposure to moisture, may be prepared into tablets after slugging.

◘   Slug

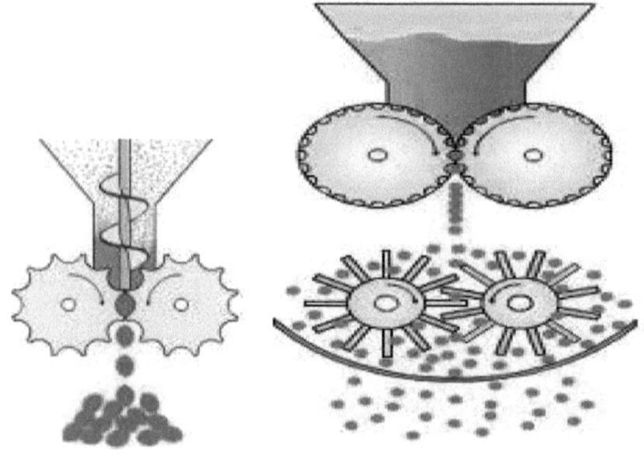

◘   **<u>Roller Compaction</u>**

◘   Instead of slugging, powder compactors may be used to increase density of powder by pressing it between rollers at 1 ton to 6 tons of pressure.

◘   Compacted material is broken up, sized and lubricated, and tablets are prepared by compression in usual manner.

◘   Roller compaction method is often preferred to slugging.

Binding agents used-methylcellulose or hydroxy methyl cellulose.

Punches and dies

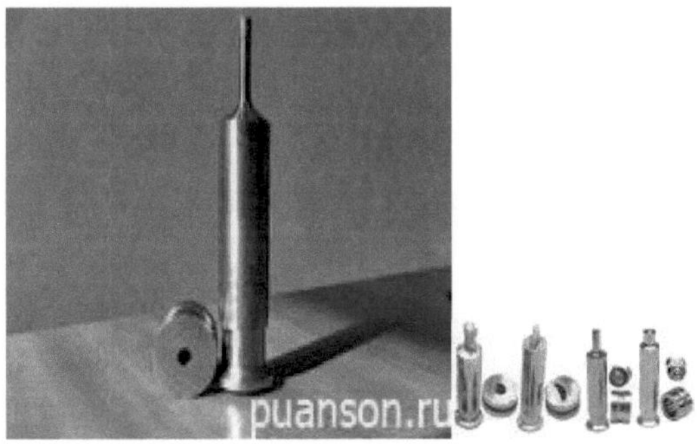

Tablet press animation

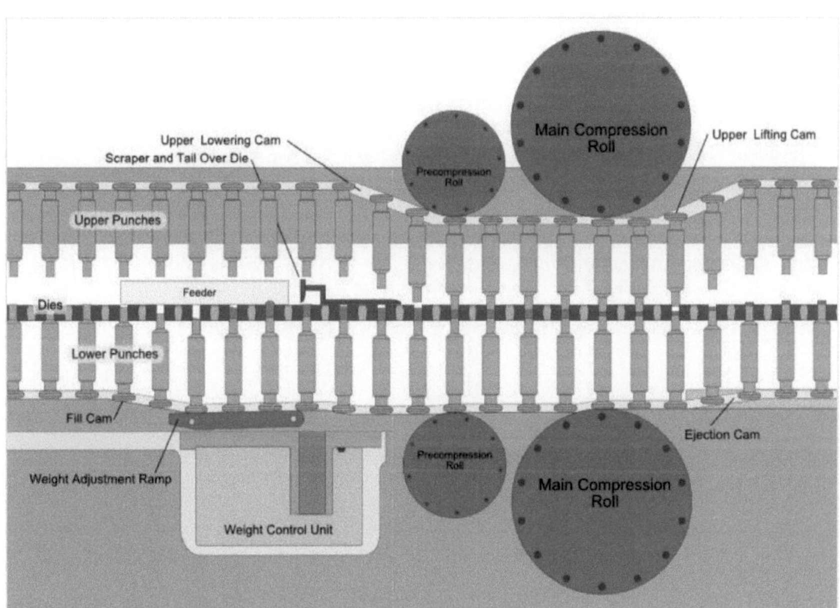

- The unused fine material may be recycled to avoid waste.

- This dry method may be used for drugs which do not compress well after wet granulation or those which are sensitive to moisture

- _Wet granulation (or wet massing)_

Wet granulation involves the massing of the powder mix using a solvent.

- The solvents used must be volatile, so that they can be removed by drying, and non-toxic.

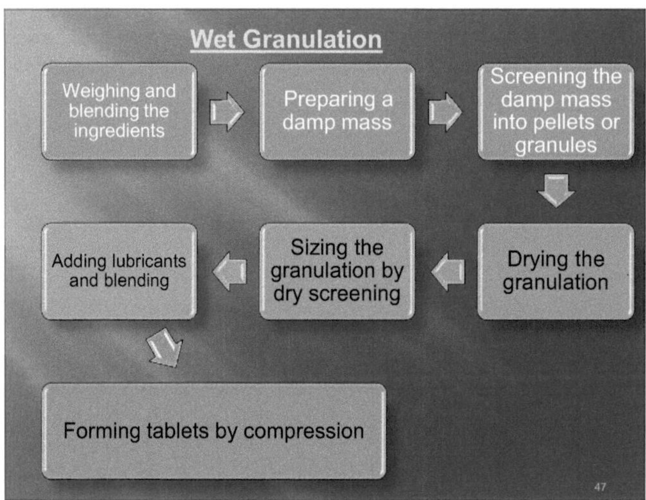

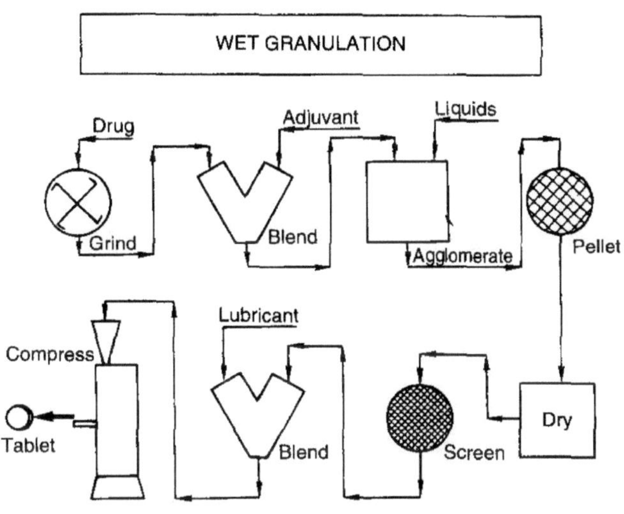

WET GRANULATION
Drug
Adjuvant
Liquids
Grind
Blend
Agglomerate
Pellet
Compress
Lubricant
Tablet
Blend
Screen
Dry

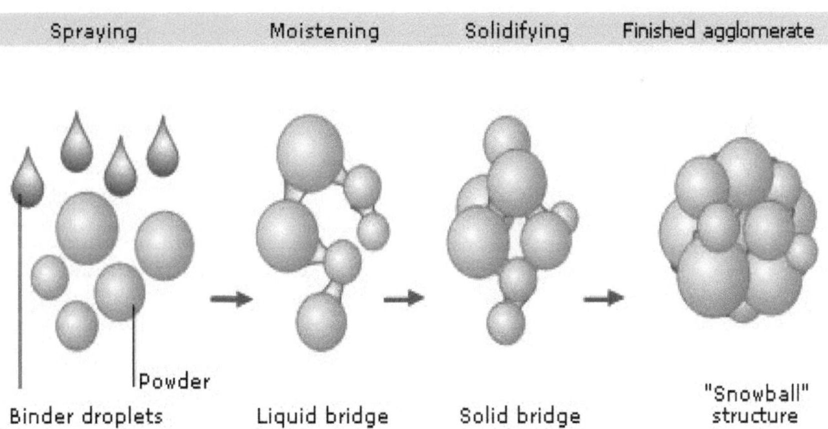

Spraying
Moistening
Solidifying
Finished agglomerate
Powder
Binder droplets
Liquid bridge
Solid bridge
"Snowball"
structure

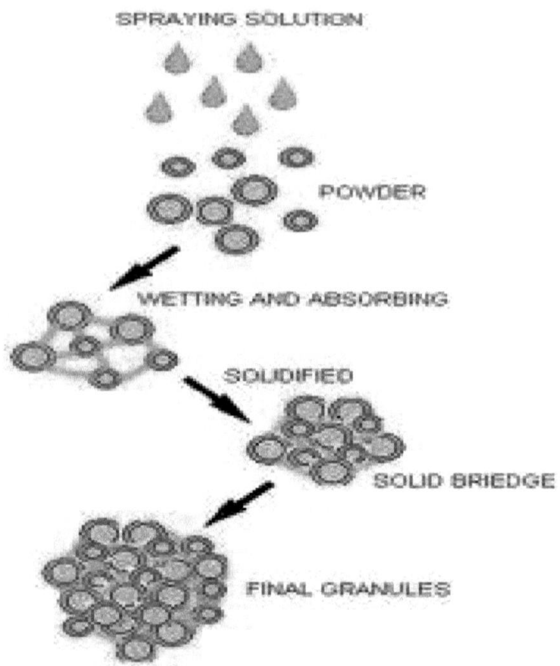

Example of granules at Infusion Stage

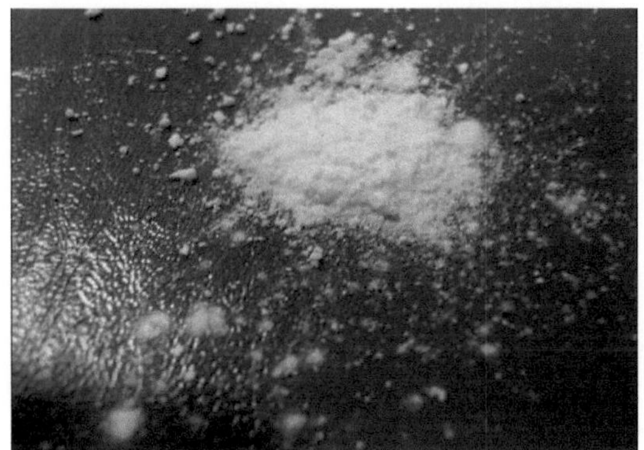

Example of chamber appearance after Stage I

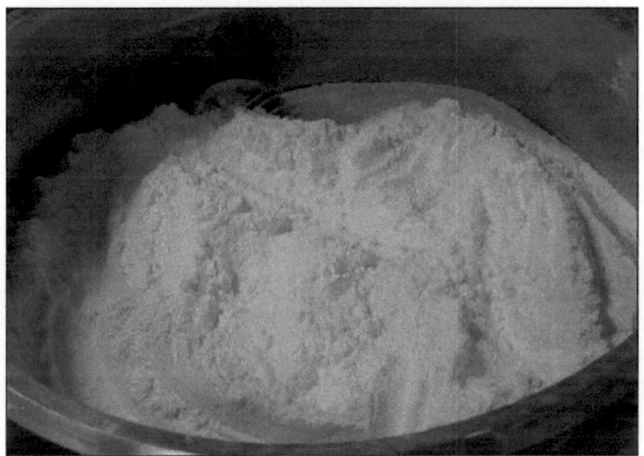

Example of end point granules at wet mass stage

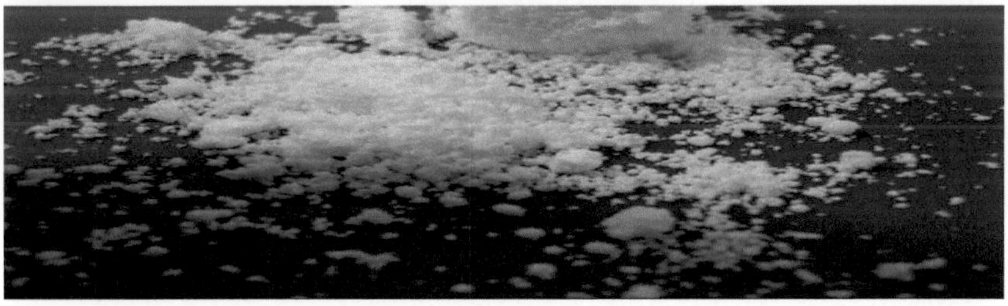

Example of end point granules at wet mass stage

46

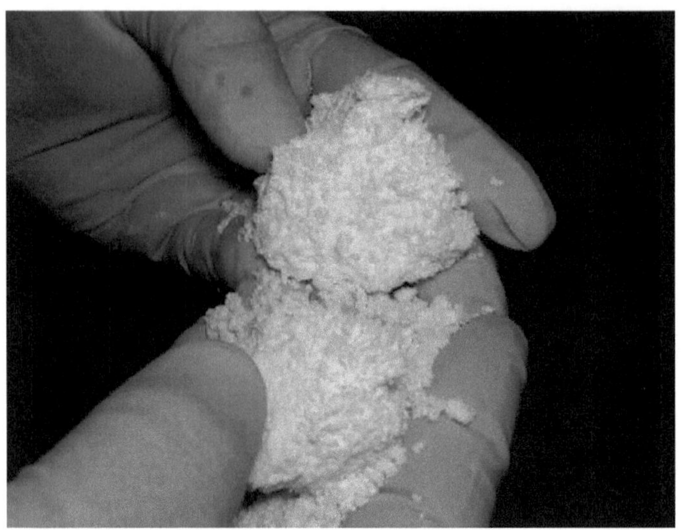

Rotary tablet pressing machine

◉   Typical solvents include

▪   water,

▪   ethanol and

▪   isopropanol either alone or in combination.

◉   The solvent may be used alone or it may contain a dissolved adhesive (also referred to as binder or binding agent) which is used to cause particle adhesion.

◉   The disadvantages of water as a solvent are that

▪   it may <u>adversely affect drug stability</u>,

▪   <u>causing hydrolysis of susceptible products</u> and

▪   It needs <u>a longer drying time</u> than organic solvents.

◉   The dry methods, adhesion of particles takes place because of applied pressure.

A compact is produced which is larger than the granule required and therefore the required size can attained by milling and sieving.

- **PHARMACEUTICAL GRANULATION EQUIPMENT**

Wet granulators

Shear granulators

High speed mixer/granulators

Fluidized bed granulators

Spray driers

Dry granulators

Sluggers

Roller compactors

Glatt WSG 120 fluid-bed granulator/dryer

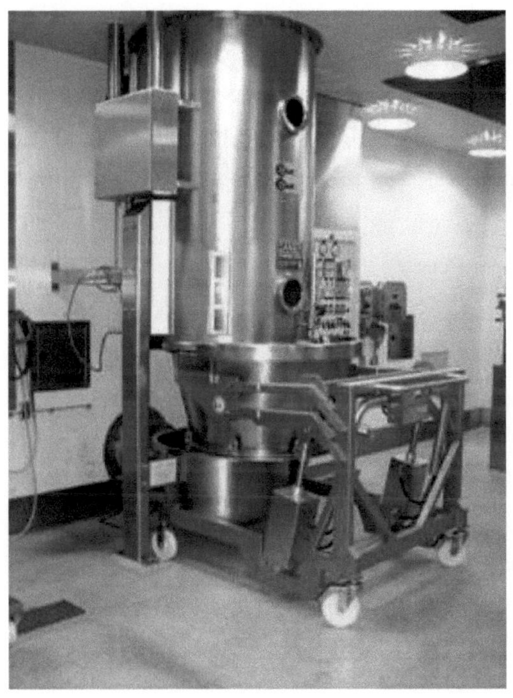

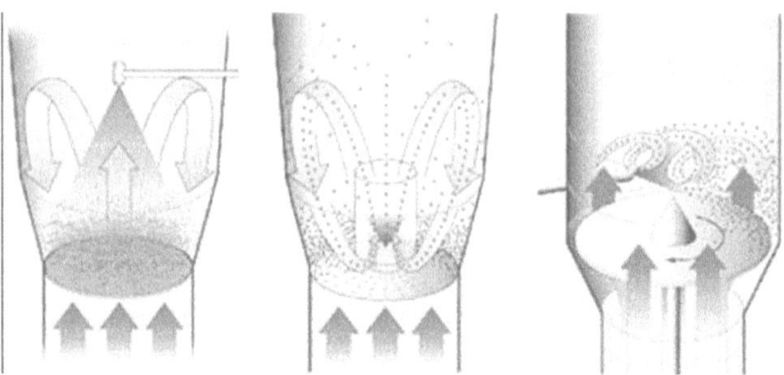

√ During the granulation process, small fine or coarse particles are converted into larger agglomerates called granules.

√ Granules enhance the uniformity of the API, increase the density of the blend, facilitate metering or volumetric dispensing, reduce dust, and improve the appearance of product.

√ The granules are formed by the following methods: solid bridges, sintering, chemical reaction, crystallization, and deposition of colloidal particles.

√ Granules are formed from the powder particles by wetting and nucleation, coalescence or growth, consolidation, and attrition or breakage.

√ Granulation technique is broadly classified into two types, dry granulation and wet granulation, with wet granulation being the most widely used granulation technique.

√ Currently available granulation technologies include roller compaction for dry granulation, and spray drying, supercritical fluid, low/high shear mixing, fluid bed granulation, and extrusion/spheronization for wet granulation.

√ Recent progress includes pneumatic dry granulation technology for dry granulation, and reverse wet granulation, steam granulation, moisture-activated dry granulation or moist granulation, thermal adhesion granulation, melt granulation, freeze granulation, foamed binder or foam granulation for wet granulation. Definitions

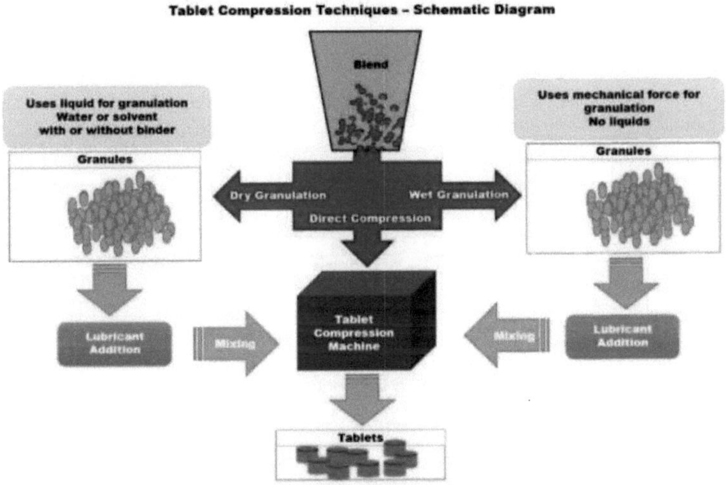

Tablet Compression Techniques – Schematic Diagram

Blend

Uses liquid for granulation
Water or solvent
with or without binder

Uses mechanical force for
granulation
No liquids

Granules

Granules

Dry Granulation

Wet Granulation

Direct Compression

Lubricant
Addition

Mixing

Tablet
Compression
Machine

Mixing

Lubricant
Addition

Tablets

Schematic diagram of tablet compression techniques

The type of process selection requires thorough knowledge of physicochemical properties of the drug, excipients, required flow and release properties, etc. Granulation technologies like roller compaction, spray drying, supercritical fluid, low/high shear mixing, fluid bed granulation, extrusion/spheronization, etc. have been successful for many decades in the preparation of various pharmaceutical dosage forms. Pharmaceutical granulation technology continues to change, and various improved, modified, and novel techniques and technologies have been made available along the course. The aim of this review is to give the reader a glimpse of the latest techniques and technologies with regard to pharmaceutical granulation. Subsequently, this review gives a short description about each development along with its significance and limitations, which are summarized in Table 1.

Table 1

Summary of recent progresses in granulation techniques and technologies

Techniques/ technologies	Description	Granule Characteristics	Merits	Limitations	Equipment
Pneumatic dry granulation	• Dry granulation • Mild Compaction and pneumatic classificatio n	√ Porous, highly compressi ble √ Taste masking √ Fast disintegrat ion √ Release time modificati on	↑ Drug loading √ Thermolabile and moisture sensitive drugs ↑ Product stability ↓ Cost and waste	X Recycled granule quality X Segregati on potential X Friability	√ Roller compactio n with air stream or vacuum
Reverse wet granulation	• Wet granulation • Water or solvent is granulating liquid	√ Uniform wetting √ Uniform erosion	↓ Particle size √ Spherical shape √ Poorly water soluble drugs	X Larger particle size$^{\perp}$ X Lower porosity X Many problems similar to conventio nal wet granulatio n	√ High speed mixer
Steam granulation	• Wet granulation • Steam is granulating liquid	↑ Diffusionr ate ↑ Uniform distributio n ↑ Surface area √ Spherical shape	√ Eco-friendly √ Sterility Process time √ No solvent use √ No health hazards	X Local over heating/w etting X High energy inputs X Thermola bile drugs X Limited binders	√ High speed mixer with steam generator/ regulator

Moisture-Activated Dry Granulati(	• Wet granulation 1-4% water is granulating liquid and moisture-absorbing material	√ Uniform size ↑ Flowability ↑ Compressibility	√ Less energy input √ No drying process √ Wide applicability √ Continuous processing ↓ Shorter process time Process variables	X Moisture sensitive drugs X Impossible high drug loading X Limited absorbents	√ High-shear mixer coupled with a sprayer
Thermal adhesion granulation	• Wet granulation • Low water/solvent is granulating liquid and heating at 30-130 °C	√ Flowability √ Friability Tensile strength	↑ Drug loading √ No drying process Dust	X High energy inputs X Thermolabile and moisture sensitive drugs X Limited binders	√ Tumble blender or similar equipment coupled with heating system
Melt granulation	• Wet granulation • Meltable binder as granulating liquid, heating at 50–90 ◦C	√ Possible modified release ↑ Dissolution	√ No water or solvent √ No drying process ↓ Energy input ↓ Cost and process time √ Water sensitive drugs	X Thermolabile drugs X Limited binders	√ High shear mixer √ Fluidized bed
Freeze granulation	• Wet granulation • Spray freezing and subsequent freeze drying for slurry or	√ Uniform size √ Flowability √ Spherical shape	↑ Granule homogeneity √ Thermolabile drugs √ Granule density control	X Limited solvent medium X Only suitable for conversion of liquid	√ Spray freezer coupled with freeze dryer

	suspensions		↓ Material waste	slurry or suspension to granules	
Foam granulation	• Wet granulation • Foam as granulating liquid	√ Uniform binder distribution √ No over wetting ↑ Surface area	↓ Water requirement No spray nozzle use √ Low water required ↓ Cost and process time √ Water sensitive drugs	X Moisture sensitive drugs X Limited binders	√ High shear mixer or fluidized bed granulator coupled with foam generator/ regulator

↓ reduced or decreased; ↑ increased or high; √ possibility or suitability or availability; X Unsuitable or not applicable. ⊥ at lower binder concentration.

Recent progress in dry granulation

Dry granulation could be achieved either by roller compaction or by slugging. The two different types are illustrated in the schematic diagram. There has not been much progress in the dry granulation technique and technology in comparison to wet granulation, except for one important innovation known as pneumatic dry granulation technology developed by Atacama LabsOy (Helsinki, Finland), which is described below. The description of its significance and limitations are summarized in Table 1.

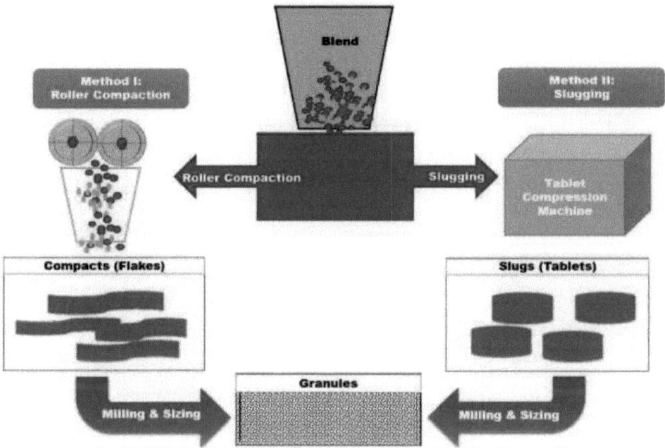

Schematic diagram of dry granulation and two different techniques. Method I is roller compaction and Method II is slugging.

Pneumatic Dry Granulation (PDG)

Pneumatic dry granulation (PDG), an innovative dry granulation technology, utilizes roller compaction together with a proprietary air classification method to produce granules with extraordinary combination of flowability and compressibility. In this method, granules are produced from powder particles by initially applying mild compaction force by roller compactor to produce a compacted mass comprising a mixture of fine particles and granules. The fine particles and/or smaller granules are separated from the intended size granules in a fractioning chamber by entraining in a gas stream (pneumatic system), whereas the intended size granules pass through the fractioning chamber to be compressed into tablets. The entrained fine particles and/or small granules are then transferred to a device such as a cyclone and are either returned to the roller compactor for immediate re-processing (recycling or recirculation process) or placed in a container for reprocessing later to achieve the granules of desired size. The schematic diagram of this process is represented below.

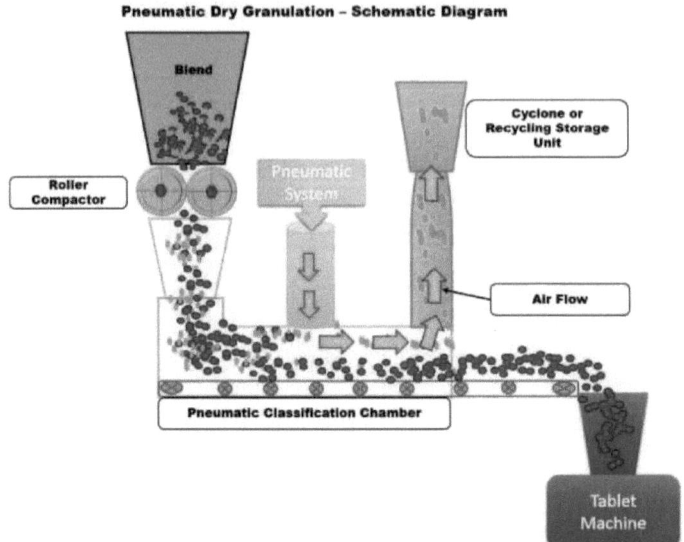

Schematic diagram of pneumatic dry granulation

PDG technology could successfully be used to produce good flowing granules for any formulations that produce compacts with a tensile strength of ~ 0.5 MPa. Also, this technology enables the use of high drug loads of up to 70-100%, because sufficient flowability could be achieved even at lower roll compaction forces (lower solid fractions) compared to usual roller compaction. In addition to these, this technology avails various other benefits such as faster processing speed, low cost, little or no material wastage, low dust exposure due to the closed nature of this unit, etc. However, the influence of recycling on the granule quality, suitability with low dose formulations, friability, etc. remains a major issues regarding this technology. The description of its significance and limitations are summarized in Table 1.

Recent progress in wet granulation

Wet granulation is the widely used technique and the granules are produced by wet massing of the excipients and API with granulation liquid with or without binder. The steps involved in conventional wet granulation technique could be seen in Fig. 4. Wet granulation has witnessed various technical and technological innovations such as steam granulation, moisture-activated dry granulation or moist granulation, thermal adhesion granulation, melt granulation, freeze granulation, foamed binder or foam granulation, and reverse wet granulation. The significance and limitations of the recent wet granulation techniques and technologies are summarized in Table 1.

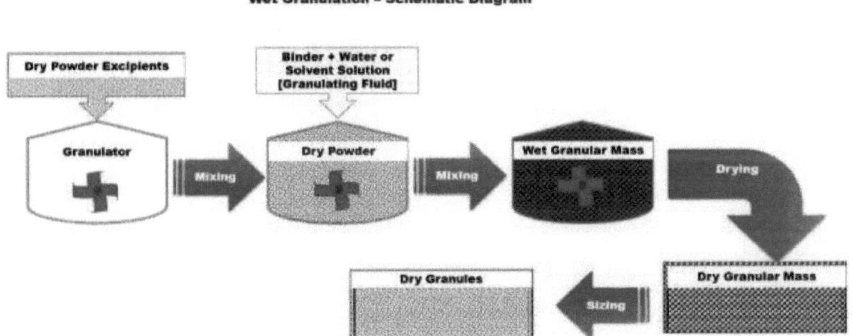

Schematic diagram of conventional wet granulation

Reverse wet granulation

Reverse wet granulation or reverse-phase wet granulation is a new development in the wet granulation technique that involves the immersion of the dry powder formulation into the binder liquid followed by controlled breakage to form granules. According to this invention, the binder solution was prepared initially and the dry powder excipients were added to the binder solution under mixing in granulator. Alternatively, the drug was mixed with a solution of hydrophilic polymer and/or binder to form a drug-polymer/binder slurry as a granulating fluid. Granules were then formed by immersing a mixture of other dry excipients into the drug-polymer/binder slurry. The resulted wet granules were milled after drying. The granules produced by this process were found to have good flow and handling characteristics like those produced with wet granulation process. In addition, tablets formed from these granules eroded more uniformly during dissolution testing as compared to usual wet granulation technique. The schematic diagram of this process is presented in Fig. 5.

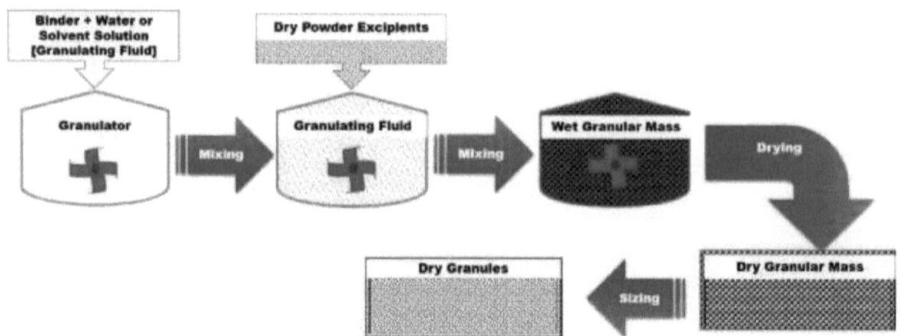

Schematic diagram of reverse wet granulation

Controlled breakage was proposed to be the predominant granule formation mechanisms in reverse wet granulation technique. It is purported that this technique improves the dissolution characteristics of the poorly water-soluble drugs by allowing uniform distribution of the binder that acts as a wetting agent and enable adequate wetting of the drug substance during granulation. It also increases the chances of adequate and uniform contact between the drug and hydrophilic polymer for better dissolution. These improved granule characteristics result in even erosion of tablets during dissolution.

The advantages of this technique over conventional wet granulation include small and spherical-shaped granules with improved flow properties, uniform wetting and erosion of the granules. This technique could be suitable for poorly water-soluble drugs because of the intimate association between a drug and the polymer. Usability of currently available equipment such as high speed mixer is another merit of this technique. However, this technique produced granules with a greater mass mean diameter and lower intragranular porosity when compared to the conventional wet granulation at lower binder concentrations.

Steam Granulation

In steam granulation as a new wet granulation technique, water steam is used as binder instead of traditional liquid water as granulation liquid. It shows the schematic diagram of steam granulation. Steam, at its pure form is transparent gas, and provides a higher diffusion rate into the powder and a more favorable thermal balance during the drying step. After condensation of the steam, water forms a hot thin film on the powder particles, requiring only a small amount of extra energy for its elimination, and evaporates more easily.[13,14]

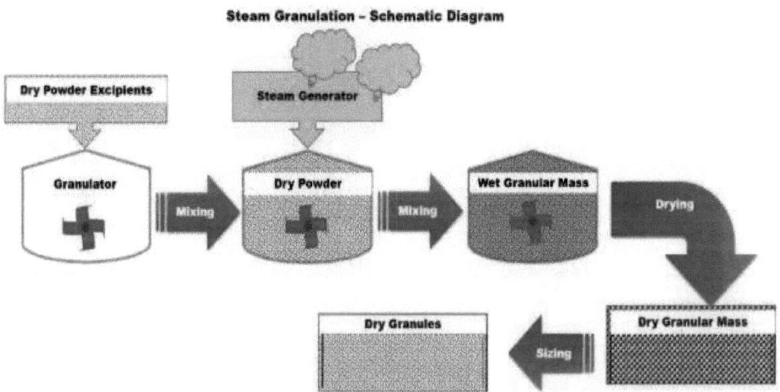

Schematic diagram of steam granulation

The advantages of this process include the higher ability of the steam to distribute uniformly and diffuse into the powder particles, production of spherical granules with larger surface area, and shorter processing time ecofriendly (no involvement of organic solvents). An equipment such as high-shear mixer coupled with a steam generator would be enough for this technique. However, this method requires high energy inputs for steam generation. Besides, this process is not suitable for all binders and is sensitive to thermolabile drugs. The granules produced by this process have higher dissolution rate due to increased surface area of the granules compared to conventional wet granulation process.

Moisture-Activated Dry Granulation (MADG)

This technique is a variation of conventional wet granulation technique. It uses very little water to activate a binder and initiate agglomeration. This technique involves two steps, 1) wet agglomeration of the powder particles, and 2) moisture absorption or distribution. Agglomeration is facilitated by adding a small amount of water, usually less than 5% (1-4% preferably), to the mixture of drug, binder and other excipients. The two steps of this MADG are presented below. Agglomeration takes place when the granulating fluid (water) activates the binder. Once the agglomeration is achieved, moisture-absorbing material such as microcrystalline cellulose, silicon dioxide, etc. is added to facilitate the absorption of excess moisture. The moisture absorbents absorb the moisture from the agglomerates, resulting in moisture redistribution within the powder mixture, leading to relatively dry granule mixture. During this moisture redistribution process, some of the agglomerates remain intact in size without change, while some larger agglomerates may break leading to more uniform particle size distribution. It does not require an expensive drying step.

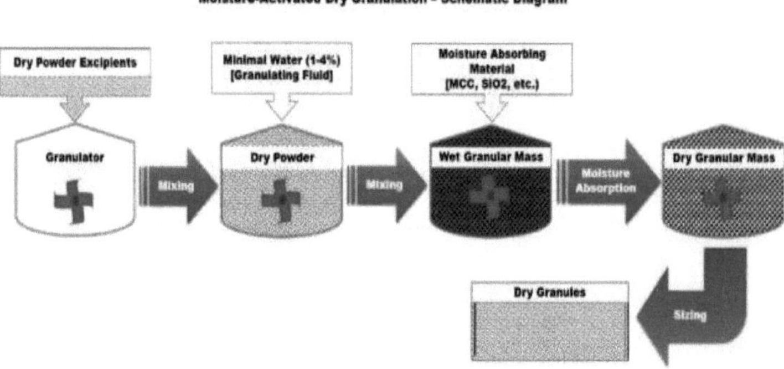

Schematic diagram of moisture-activated dry granulation

The process does not lead to larger lumps formation since the amount of water used is very small compared to usual wet granulation. The particle size of the agglomerates is mainly accounted to be in the range of 150-500 µm. This technique is also known as "moist granulation technique" leading to confusions with the use of appropriate terminology. Some authors believe that dry granulation involves the use of a roller compaction or a slugging step followed by milling to obtain granules. However, this technique did not use either of those steps. Besides, given that this technique utilizes a small amount of water, the use of the term "dry granulation" would be inappropriate. Therefore, the authors believe that "moist granulation" would be an appropriate terminology for this technique. In either case, the technique is the same and this review uses the terminology "Moisture-Activated Dry Granulation (MADG)" coined by the inventors of this technique in 1987.

The application of MADG to an immediate-release and controlled-release dosage forms showed the advantages of wet granulation such as increased particle size, better flow and compressibility. Additional advantages of this technique include wide applicability, time efficiency and less energy input, and involvement of few process variables with suitability of continuous process. However, this technique could not be used for the preparation of granules that require high drug load and for moisture sensitive drugs and hygroscopic drugs due to stability and processing problems associated with these types of drugs. A high-shear mixer coupled with a sprayer would be a suitable equipment for the MADG process. An ideal machine should be equipped with efficient impellers, blades, and choppers to allow good mass movement and proper mixing of the granulation mass.

Thermal Adhesion Granulation (TAG)

Wei-Ming Pharmaceutical Company (Taipei, Taiwan) has developed this technique, and the thermal adhesion granulation, analogous to moist granulation, utilizes addition of a small amount of granulation liquid and heat for agglomeration. This is clearly presented in Figure as a schematic diagram. Unlike moisture activated dry granulation which uses water alone as granulation liquid, this process uses both water and solvent as granulation liquid. In addition to this, heat is used to facilitate the granulation process. In this process, the drug and excipient mixture is heated to a temperature range of 30–130 °C in a closed system under tumble rotation to facilitate the agglomeration of the powder particles. This technique eliminates the drying process due to the addition of low amount of granulation liquid, which is mostly consumed by the powder particles during agglomeration. Granules of the required particle size can be obtained after cooling and sieving.

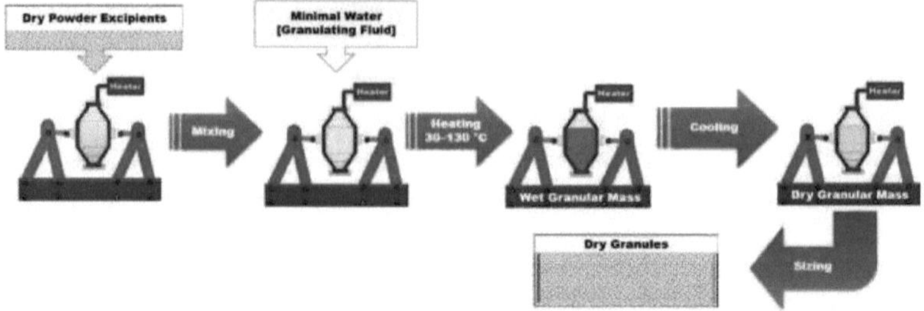

Schematic diagram of thermal adhesion granulation

This technique is quite simple and convenient with low moisture and binder contents in a closed system for preparing highly compressible materials or for modifying the poor characteristics of excipients. Besides, this technique provides granules with better particle size, good flow properties and high tensile strength that could be directly compressed into tablets with adequate hardness and low friability. The limitations of this technique are requirement of considerably high energy inputs and special equipment for heat generation and regulation. This technique is not suitable for all binders and is sensitive to thermolabile drugs.

Melt granulation

Melt granulation or thermoplastic granulation is a technique that facilitates the agglomeration of powder particles using meltable binders, which melts or softens at relatively low temperature (50–90 °C). Figure represents the schematic diagram of melt granulation. Cooling of the agglomerated powder and the consequent solidification of the molten or soften binder complete the granulation process. Low melting binders can be added to the granulation process either in the form of solid particles that melt during the process (melt-in procedure or in situ melt granulation) or in the form of molten liquid, optionally containing the dispersed drug (spray-on or pump-on procedure), which displays a variety of options to design final granular properties. More specifically, the melt-in procedure of melt granulation process includes heating a mixture of drug, binder and other excipients to a temperature within or above the melting range of the binder. On the contrary, the spray-on procedure encompasses spraying of a molten binder, optionally containing the drug, onto the heated powders.

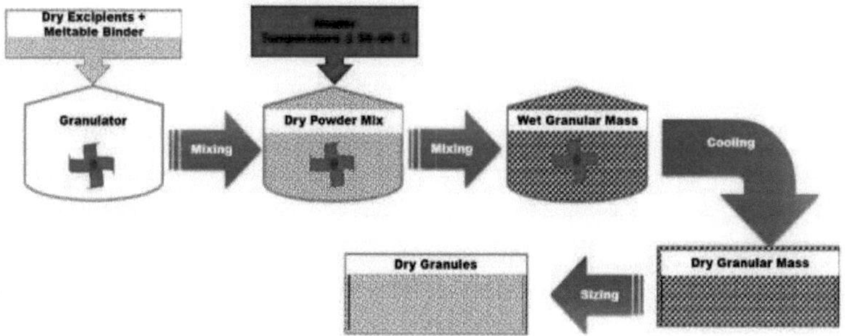

Schematic diagram of melt granulation

Melt granulation is an appropriate alternative to other wet granulation techniques which are used for water sensitive materials. Moreover, in comparison with the conventional wet granulation process, it proposes several advantages. Generally, organic or aqueous solvents are not demanded for the melt granulation process, hence the environmental requirements of organic solvent capture and recycling are eliminated, while the absence of water excludes the wetting and drying phases, making the entire process less energy- and time-consuming. Melt granulation method could be efficiently applied in order to enhance the stability of moisture sensitive drug and further to improve the poor physical properties of the drug substance. The major drawback of this process is the need of high temperature during the process, which can cause degradation and/or oxidative instability of the ingredients, especially of the thermolabile drugs.

The binders used for this process could be either hydrophilic or hydrophobic. The selection of a meltable binder with a hydrophilic/hydrophobic feature is critical factor for the dissolution behavior of the drugs. The equipments that could be used for melt granulation are high-shear mixer and fluidized bed granulator. Interest in melt granulation has increased in recent years, owing to the numerous advantages of this technique over conventional wet granulation process.

Freeze granulation

Freeze granulation technology, spray freezing and subsequent freeze drying, involves spraying droplets of a liquid slurry or suspension into liquid nitrogen followed by freeze-drying of the frozen droplets. By spraying a powder suspension into liquid nitrogen, the drops are instantly frozen into granules, and in the subsequent freeze drying process, the granules are dried by sublimation of ice without any segregation effects. This process yields spherical free-flowing granules that could be formed by using both water based and solvent based slurries. The significance of this technology is that the structure and homogeneity of the particles in the slurry or suspension are retained in the granules. Although various kinds of material in dispersed form can be granulated using this technology, it is suitable for the preparation of fine powder mixes with proper additives for subsequent processing.

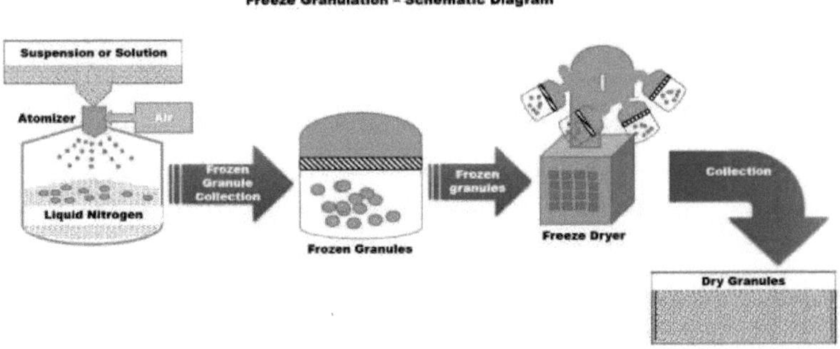

Schematic diagram of freeze granulation

This technology could be useful for the preparation of granules that needs to be prepared from suspensions whose particle size and homogeneity need to be preserved. Eventually, re-dispersible parenteral formulations, nanomaterials, solid self-emulsifying drug delivery systems, etc. could benefit from this technology given its ability to maintain size and homogeneity. The suspension quality always determines and reflects the granule quality in terms of homogeneity. In pharmaceutical industry, the low-temperature and soft freeze drying has vital advantage to minimize damage of organic compounds and improve stability and/or solubility. According to PowderPro AB, compared with spray drying, freeze granulation obviously produces protein particles with light and porous characteristics, and making powders with superior aerosol performance due to favorable aerodynamic properties.

The major advantages of this process include ability to control the granule density through the solid content of the suspension, preparation of granules with no cavities, a high degree of granule homogeneity due to the absence of migration of small particles and/or binder molecules, use of heat sensitive compounds due to mild drying procedure, high product yield due to low waste of material, and possibility of recycling organic solvents. Although organic solvents with suitable freezing point (-25 to +10 °C) can be used, water as medium is preferred in this process, which could be a limiting criteria given the poor solubility of various drugs and processing excipients. Originally, this process was developed by Swedish Ceramic Institute in the late 1980. Currently, PowderPro AB, the spinoff company (year 2000) from Swedish Ceramic Institute, develops, manufactures, markets, and sells equipment for freeze granulation.

Foam granulation

Foam granulation or foamed binder granulation technology, analogous to spray agglomeration, involves the addition of liquid/aqueous binder as foam instead of spraying or pouring liquid onto the powder particles. This shows the schematic diagram of this technology. This foam binder technology was first introduced by Dow Chemical Company (Midland, MI) in 2003 for delivering aqueous binder systems in high shear and fluid bed wet granulation applications. A foam generator can be installed in the binder solution tank with high-shear granulator or fluid bed granulator to introduce the binder as foam rather than spraying or pouring in binder onto the moving powder particles. Adding the binder solution as foam rather than a spray eliminates the problems of inconsistent and unpredictable binder distribution that can affect tablet hardness and drug release.

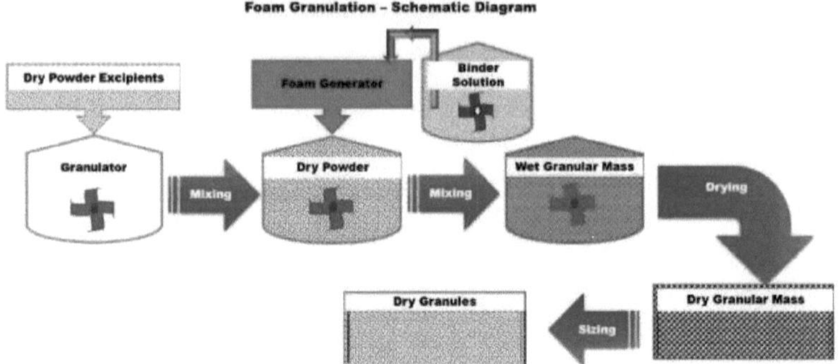

Schematic diagram of foam granulation

The surface area and volume of the foamed binder/water are phenomenally high compared to the sprayed water. This technology exploits the characteristics of the foamed binder to successfully improve the distribution of binder onto the powder particles, even at a binder amount lower than that required in the conventional spray granulation method. Besides, the sprayed liquid droplets have a low spread-to-soak ratio, which means they tend to soak into powders and cause overwetting rather than spreading on the surface of the particles, requiring high levels of water and binder, and eventually drying to remove excess water. On the contrary, foamed binders have a high spread-to-soak ratio, and because of this the binders are coated onto the particles rather than soaked, leading to less amount of binder and more consistent binder distribution. These factors improve the reproducibility and shorten the processing time. Most importantly, this technology eliminates the spray nozzles and its related processing variables and clogging problems.

In addition to the above-mentioned advantages, this technology would prove useful for high potent/low dose drug formulations due to its ability to distribute drugs evenly. Due to the involvement of low amount of water and short process time, water sensitive formulations could also be prepared using this technology in addition to immediate release and controlled release formulations. Standard equipment such as high/low shear mixer, fluid bed granulator, etc. could be used for this technology in association with a foam generator. Although this technology merits in myriad ways, further understanding of foam quality, process parameters, equipment, flow patterns, mixing behavior, etc. needs to be explored. Besides, the regulatory approval would be a huge hurdle that needs to be overcome.

Conclusion

Technical and technological innovations that improve and ease existing processes could contribute to improved processability and quality of the product formulations in addition to a substantial impact on the product development, time and economy. Obviously, the pharmaceutical granulation techniques and technologies have improved over the years. Nevertheless, efficient and cost-effective manufacturing methods have always been the keen interest of the pharmaceutical industries, which catapults the research and development of new and improved technologies by the interdisciplinary scientists of pharmaceutical companies globally. During the formulation development, each drug substance poses a unique challenge that must be taken into consideration at the process selection stage by the formulation development scientists. Each technique has its own merits and limitations, and the type of technique and technology selection requires thorough knowledge of physicochemical properties of the drug, excipients, required flow and release properties, etc. in addition to the granulation techniques and technologies itself. This review discussed the recent developments in granulation technology for conventional release dosage formulations only. Nonetheless, when it comes to orally disintegrating tablets (ODTs), new technologies like Orasolv®, Durasolv®, Wowtab®, Flashtab®, Zydis®, Flashdose®, Oraquick®, Lyoc®, Advatab®, Frosta®, Quick-Disc® and Nanomelt® have been introduced by various pharmaceutical companies for the production of ODTs, which is beyond the scope of this review. In the pharmaceutical industry, although various technologies have been introduced from time to time, only few have emerged as successful for real time utilization due to different kinds of hurdles such as manufacturing efficiency, economy, regulatory issues, etc. The author's opinion is that the new techniques and technologies discussed in this review would need enhancements in terms of equipment, process, etc. before being industrialized successfully. Nevertheless, these could provide a platform for further technological innovation.

References:

1. Kamble N. et al Innovations in Tablet Coating Technology: A Review. International Journal of Applied Biology and Pharmaceutical Technology, 2011, 214 – 218

2. Invensys Eurotherm. The Tablet Coating Process [Cited 2012 Aug. 18], Available from http://www.eurotherm.com/industries/life- sciences/applications/tablet-coating/

3. Lachman leon et al," The theory and Practice of Industrial Pharmacy" Second Edition, Forth Indian reprint, Published by Varghese Publishing House, Bombay, 1991, 346 – 372

4. Tech Tips, Aqueous Coating 101. Techceuticals Solutions for Pharma & Nutra Manufacturers since 1989 [Cited 2012 Aug. 05], Available from http://www.techceuticals.com/techtips/show_news.php?subaction=show full&id=1079300125&archive=&star

5. Marjeram J., Advancements in Continuous Tablet Coating, [Cited 2012 Feb.   13], Available from http://www.cvg.ca/Presentations/2008/OHaraOct2008presentation to2008CVGconventionR1.pdf

6. Gohel M. Tablet Coating, 2009, [Cited 2012 Feb. 23], Available from http://www.pharmainfo.net/ tablet-ruling-dosage-form-years/tablet- coating

7. Zhu J. Et al Tablet Coating. CSC Publishing, 2009, [Cited 2012 July 17],   Available from http://www.patheon.com/Portals/0/Scientific%20Papers/Published%20A rticles/tc_20 100401_0018.pdf

8. Qiao M. et al A Novel Electrostatic Dry Powder Coating Process for Pharmaceutical Dosage Forms: Immediate Release Coatings for Tablets. European Journal of Pharmaceutics and Biopharmaceutics, 2010, 304- 310

9. Pawar A. et al Advances in Pharmaceutical Coatings. International Journal of ChemTech Research, 2010, 733 – 737

10. Patentgenius, Phoqus Pharmaceutical Limited Patents. Patentgenius, 2011,   [Cited 2012 Aug. 21], Available   from http://www.patentgenius.com/assignee/PhoqusPharmaceuticals Limited.html

11.Singh P. et al Estimation of Coating Time in The Magnetically Assisted Impaction Coating Process. Elsevier, 2001, 159-167

12.Tamahane P.M. Enteric Aqueous Film Coating. Wincoat Colours & Coatings Pvt. Ltd., 2011, [Cited 2012 July 17], Available from http://www. wincoatreadymix.com/enteric-aqueous-film-coating.html

13. Pareek S., Sharad C.R. Aqueous Film Coating: Critical Aspects, Pharma Technology-Express Pharma Pulse (Special Feature), 2003.

14. GEA Niro Pharma Systems. SupercellTM Coating Technology (SCT), [Cited 2012 Feb.13],

15. Elaine S. K. Tang et al Study of Coat Quality of Tablets Coated by an On-line Supercell Coater. AAPS PharmSciTech, 2007, E92-E98

16. Breakthrough Tablet Coater Unveiled by Niro, 2004, [Cited 2012 July 17], Available from http://www.in- pharmatechnologist.com/Processing/Breakthrough-tablet-coater-unveiled-by-Niro

17. Shah A. Coating Tablet Defects: The Cause and the Remedies, 2011, [Cited 2012 July 17], Available from http://vikramthermo.blogspot.in/2011/06/picking-and sticking.html

18. Picta R. Problems associated with Tablet Manufacturing, 2011, [Cited 2012 July 17], Available from http://www.pharmainfo.net/rajapicta1023/blog/problems-associated-tablet-manufacturing

19. Cunningham C. Investigation of a new Coating Process for the Application of Enteric Coatings to Small Tablet Samples, Poster Reprint AAPS Annual Meeting and exposition, 2005 [cited 2012 Feb. 13], Available from http://www.niroinc.com/ html/pharma/phpdfs/new_coating_ process

20. Behzadi S. Innovations in Coating Technology, Recent Patents on drug Delivery & Formulations, 2008; 209 – 230

21. Shah A. Coating Tablet Defects: The Cause and the Remedies. Coating Polymers, 2011, [Cited 2012 Aug. 05],

22. Tablet Defects, 2012, [Cited 2012 March 12], Available from http://www .scribd.com/doc/41292307/ Tablet-Defects

23. Magnetically Assisted Impaction Mixing, 2011, [Cited 2012 July 17], Available   from http://www.ndcee.ctc.com/technologies/Coatings- Surface_Preparation/Coatings_In organic/Magnetically_Assisted_Impaction_Mixing.pdf

24. Tousey M. Tablet Coating Basics. CSC Publishing, [Cited 2012 Feb. 13], Available from http://www.dipharma.com/TC_20050401_20.pdf

25. Thakral S. K. and Gupta V. Advances in Tablet Coating, 1998, [Cited 2012   Feb.   23],

26. Allen, LV, Nicholas G, Ansel HC. Ansel's Pharmaceutical Dosage Forms and Drug Delivery Systems (9th ed.), Lippincott Williams & Wilkins, 2011(Latest edition).

27. Sinko PJ. Martin's Physical Pharmacy and Pharmaceutical Sciences (6th ed.), Lippincott Williams & Wilkins; 2010(Latest edition)

28. Aulton, M.E. Pharmaceutics: The Science of dosage form design, (2nd ed.), Churchill Livingstone, (Latest edition).

<h1 style="text-align:center"><u>Chapter 4.</u></h1>

<h2 style="text-align:center"><u>Tablets Dosage Form</u></h2>

<u>Objectives</u>

- To know the basic information about tablet dosage form

- To understand the various types of tablet dosage form

- To explain the development of Formulation

- To Understand the Quality standards and compendial requirements

Introduction

▫ Tablets are solid dosage forms usually prepared with the aid of suitable pharmaceutical excipients.

▫ They may vary in size, shape, weight, hardness, thickness, disintegration and dissolution characteristics.

▫ Most tablets are used in the oral administration of drugs.

▫ Many of these are prepared with colorants and coatings of various types.

▫ Tablets are prepared primarily by compression, with limited number prepared by molding

▫ Compressed tablets are manufactured with tablet machines capable of <u>exerting great pressure</u> in compacting the powdered or granulated material

▫ Molded tablets are prepared on a large –scale by tablet machinery or on a small –scale by manually forcing dampened powder material into a mold from which the formed tablet is then ejected and allowed to dry.

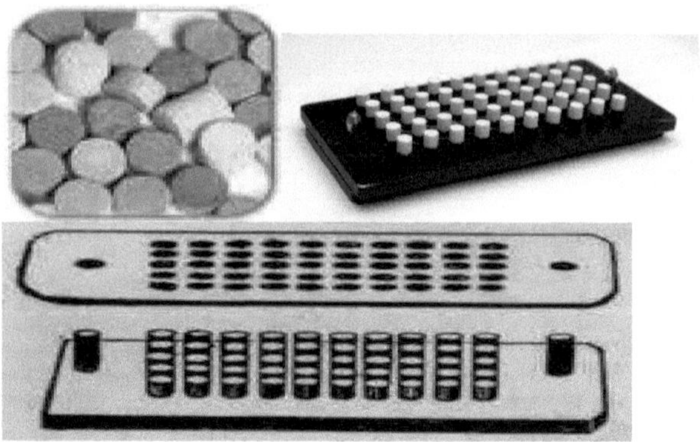

- Some tablets are scored or grooved, which allows them to be easily broken into two or more parts.

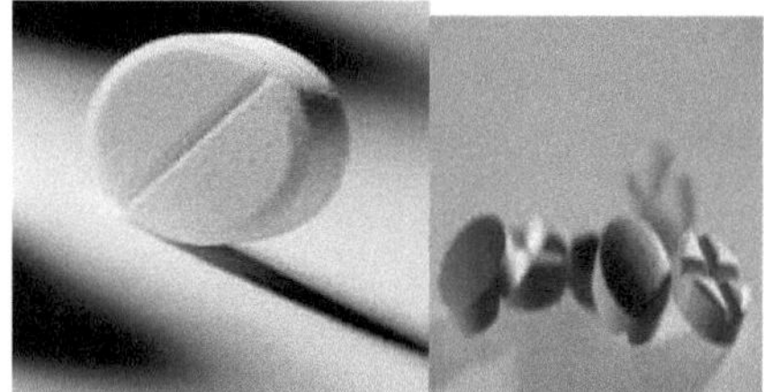

- Tablets that are not scored are not intended to be broken or cut by the patient since they may have special coatings and/or drug release features that would be compromised by altering the tablets physical integrity.

Different types of Tablets

- **(A) Tablets ingested orally:**

  - 1. Compressed tablet, e.g. Paracetamol tablet

  - 2. Multiple compressed tablet

  - 3. Repeat action tablet

  - 4. Delayed release tablet, e.g. Enteric coated Bisacodyl tablet

- □   5. Sugar coated tablet, e.g. Multivitamin tablet

- □   6. Film coated tablet, e.g. Metronidazole tablet

- □   7. Chewable tablet, e.g. Antacid tablet

- ■ **(B) Tablets used in oral cavity**:

- □   1. Buccal tablet, e.g. Vitamin-c tablet

- □   2. Sublingual tablet, e.g. Vicks Menthol tablet

- □   3. Troches or lozenges

- □   4. Dental cone

- ■ **(c) Tablets administered by other route:**

- ■   1. Implantation tablet

- ■   2. Vaginal tablet, e.g. Clotrimazole tablet

- ■ **(D) Tablets used to prepare solution**:

- □   1. Effervescent tablet, e.g. Dispirin tablet (Aspirin)

- □   2. Dispersing tablet, e.g. Enzyme tablet (Digiplex)

- □   3. Hypodermic tablet

- □   4. Tablet triturates e.g. Enzyme tablet (Digiplex)

- ■ <u>**Types of tablets**</u>

- ■ <u>1.Compressed tablets</u>

- ■ In addition to the medicinal agent or agents, compressed tablets usually contain a number of pharmaceutical adjuncts.

- □   <u>Diluents or fillers</u> —which add the necessary bulk to a formulation to prepare tablets of the desired size.

- □   <u>Binders or adhesives-</u> which promote adhesion of the particles of the formulation allowing a granulation to be prepared and maintaining the integrity of the final tablet.

- Disintegrants-

□ which promote breakup of the tablets after administration to smaller particles for ready drug availability.

□ Antiadherents, glidants, lubricants –

□ which enhance the flow of the material into the tablet dies,

□ minimize wear of the punches and dies,

□ prevent fill material from sticking to the punches and dies and

□ produce tablets with a sheen.

- After compression, tablets may be coated with various materials.

- Tablets for

□ Oral,

□ Buccal,

□ Sublingual,

□ Vaginal administration may be prepared by compression

2. Multiple Compressed Tablets

- Prepared by subjecting the fill material to more than a single compression.

- The result may be a <u>multiple-layer tablet</u> or <u>a tablet within a tablet</u>, the inner tablet being the core and outer portion being the shell.

- <u>Layered tablets are prepared by initial compaction of a portion of fill material in a die followed by additional fill material and compression to form two-or three layered tablets, depending on the number of separate fills.</u>

- Each layer may contain a different medicinal agent, separated for reasons of

- chemical or physical incompatibility,

- staged drug release, or

- Simply for unique appearance of layered tablet.

- Usually, each portion of fill is a different color to produce a distinctive-looking tablet.

- In preparation of tablets within tablets, special machines are required to place the preformed core tablet precisely within the die for application of surrounding fill material.

3.Sugarcoated Tablets

- Coating is water soluble and quickly dissolves after swallowing.

- Sugar coat

  - Protects the enclosed drug from the environment

  - Provided barrier to objectionable taste or odor.

  - Enhances the appearance of compressed tablet

  - Permits imprinting of identifying manufacturer's information.

- Compressed tablets may be coated with a colored or an uncolored sugar layer.

- **Disadvantage**

- Time

- Expertise required in coating process

- Increase in size, weight, and shipping costs.

- Sugar coating may add 50% to the weight and bulk of uncoated tablet.

- **4.Film-Coated Tablets**

- Are compressed tablets <u>coated with a thin layer of a polymer</u> capable of forming a skin like film.

- Film is usually colored and has the advantage over sugarcoating in that

  - it is more durable,

  - less bulky and

  - Less time consuming to apply.

- By its composition, the coating is designed to rupture and expose the core tablet at the desired location in the gastrointestinal tract.

- **<u>5.Gelatin-coated tablets</u>**

  A recent innovation

  The innovator product, the gelcap, is a capsule shaped compressed tablet that allows the coated product to be about one-third smaller than a capsule filled with an equivalent amount of powder.

  <u>Gelatin coating facilitates swallowing.</u>

  They are more tamper evident than unsealed capsules.

- **<u>6.Enteric-coated Tablets</u>**

- They have delayed-release features.

- Are designed to pass unchanged through the stomach to the intestines, where tablets disintegrate and allow drug dissolution and absorption and /or effect.

-   Enteric coatings are employed

    when the drug substance is destroyed by gastric acid or

    are particularly irritating to the gastric mucosa or

    when by pass of stomach substantially enhances drug absorpti**on.**

<u>7. Lozenges or troches</u>

- They are disc shaped solid dosage forms containing a medicinal agent and generally a flavoring substance in a hard candy or sugar base.

- Intended to be slowly dissolved in the oral cavity, usually for local effects, although some are formulated for systemic absorption.

- **<u>8.Chewable Tablets</u>**

- Have a smooth,

- rapid disintegration when chewed or

- allowed to dissolve in the mouth,

- Have creamy base, usually of specially flavored and colored.

- Are especially useful for administration of large tablets to children and adults who have difficulty in swallowing solid dosage forms.

- Mainly prepared by Wet granulation

- Main Excipient is Mannitol (White Crystalline hexahydric alcohol) especially for moisture-sensitive drugs because mannitol is non-hygroscopic material.

- **9.Effervescent Tablets**

- Prepared by compressing granular effervescent salts that release gas when in contact with water.

- They generally contain medicinal substances that dissolve rapidly when added to water.

10.Molded tablets

- Certain tablets such as tablet triturates,

- May be prepared by molding rather than by compression.

- Resultant tablets are very soft and soluble

- Designed for rapid dissolution.

11. Tablet Triturates

- Are small,

- usually cylindrical,

- Molded or compressed tablets containing small amounts of usually potent drugs.

- Only a few tablet triturate products are available commercially, with most of these produced by tablet compression.

- Since tablet triturates must be readily and completely soluble in water, only a minimal amount of pressure is applied during their manufacture.

- A combination of sucrose and lactose is usually the diluent.

- Few tablet triturates that remain are used sublingually, such as nitroglycerin tablets.

- Pharmacists also employ tablet triturates in compounding.

- For example, triturates are inserted into capsules or dissolved in liquid to provide accurate amounts of potent drug substances.

- **12.Hypodermic Tablets**

- Are no longer available in the United States

- Were originally used by physicians in extemporaneous (not marketed product, compounding product by Pharmacist) preparation of parenteral solutions

- Required number of tablets were dissolved in a suitable vehicle, sterility attained and the injection performed.

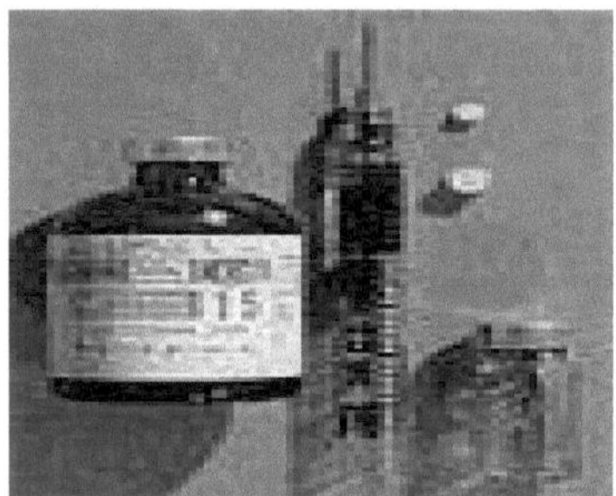

- Tablets were a convenience, since they could be easily carried in the physician's medicine bag and injections prepared to meet the needs of the individual patients.

However, the difficulty in achieving sterility and availability of prefabricated injectable products, some in disposable syringes, have eliminated the need for hypodermic tablets

13. Immediate-Release Tablets

- Are designed to disintegrate and release their medication w<u>ntegrating or Dissolving Tablets</u>

- Are characterized by disintegrating ith no special rate-controlling features, such as special coatings and other techniques.

14. Instantly Disiolving tablets dissolving in the mouth within 1 minute, some within 10 seconds

- (e.g.Claritin Reditabs [loratadine],Schering).

- Tablets of this type are designed for children and the elderly or for any patient who has difficulty in swallowing tablets.

- They liquefy on the tongue, and the patient swallows the liquid.

- Techniques used to prepare the tablets include

- lyophilization,

- Soft direct compression and other methods (Spray drying, molten method).

- Are prepared using very water-soluble excipients designed to wick water into the tablet for rapid disintegration or dissolution.

- Have stability characteristics of other solid dosage forms.

- Original fast-dissolving tablets were molded tablets for sublingual use.

- Generally consisted of active drug and lactose moistened with an alcohol-water mixture to form a paste.

- Tablets were then molded, dried, and packaged.

- For use simply placed in tongue to provide rapid onset of action for drugs such as nitroglycerin.

- Also have been used for drugs that are destroyed in GIT, such as testosterone, administered sublingually for absorption to minimize first pass effect

- New RDTs are designed for oral use by patients who have difficulty swallowing standard tablets and capsules, such as children and elderly.

Are more convenient to carry and administer than an oral liquid.

No standards that define RDT, but one possibility is dissolution in the mouth within approx 15-30 sec.

Anything slower would not be categorized as rapidly dissolving.

- For a product to dissolve instantly, it may be quite friable.

- Making it more firm and less friable may increase dissolution time.

- A balance must be achieved between friability and speed of dissolution.

- **<u>15.Extended-Release Tablets</u>**

- Sometimes called controlled release are designed to release their medication in a predetermined manner over an extended period.

- <u>17.Vaginal Tablets</u>

- Also called vaginal inserts

- They are uncoated bullet-shaped or ovoid tablets inserted into the vagina for local effects.

- Prepared by compression and shaped to fit snugly on plastic inserter devices that accompany the product.

- Contain <u>antibacterials for treatment of vaginitis caused by Haemophilus vaginalis or antifungals for treatment of vulvovaginitis candidiasis caused by candida albicans and related species</u>

- <u>Compressed Tablets</u>

- <u>Physical features are well known</u>:

- round, oblong, or unique in shape;

- thick or thin;

- Large or small in diameter.

- flat or convex,

- unscored or scored in halves, thirds, or quadrants;

- engraved or imprinted with symbol and

- code number,

- coated or uncoated,

- Colored or uncolored.

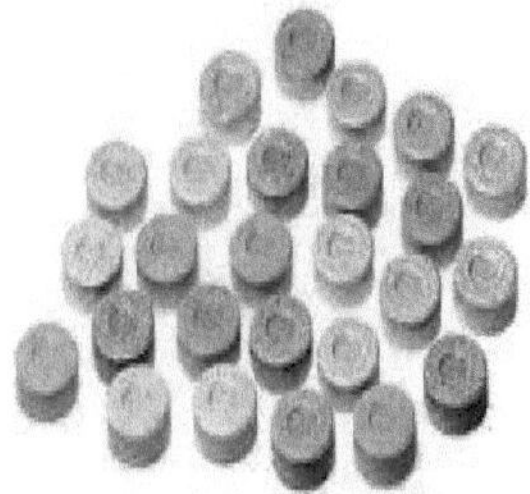

- Tablet diameters and shapes are determined by dies and punches used in compression.

- <u>Less concave the punches, flatter the tablets</u>

- <u>More concave the punches, more convex the tablets</u>

- <u>Punches with raised impressions produce recessed impressions on the tablets</u>

- Punches with recessed etchings produce tablets with raised impressions or monograms.

- Monograms may be placed on one or on both sides of a tablet, depending on the punches.

- <u>Monograms:</u>

- To mark with a design composed of one or more letters.

- Advantages of tablets:

- 1. Ease of accurate dosing

- 2. Good physical and chemical stability

- 3. Low cost

- 4. High level of patient acceptability

- 5. High convenience

Disadvantages of tablets

1. Irritant effect on GI mucosa

2. Possibility of bioavailability problems.

Advantages of tablets:

- 1. Ease of accurate dosing

- 2. Good physical and chemical stability

- 3. Low cost

- 4. High level of patient acceptability

- 5. High convenience

Three basic methods:

- Wet granulation

- Dry granulation

- Direct compression

- <u>**Wet Granulation**</u>

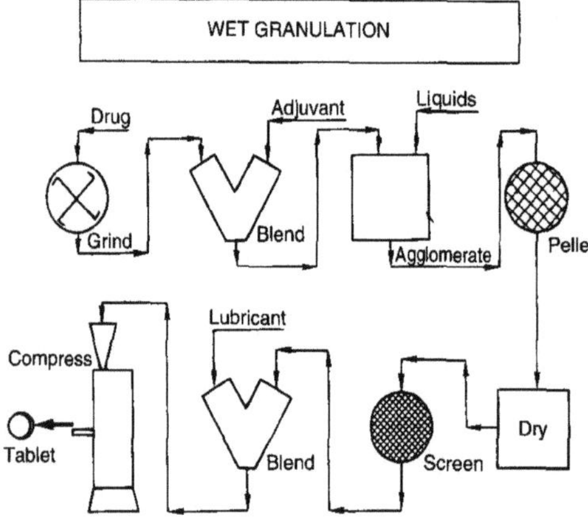

- As lower punch drops, feed shoe filled with granulation from hopper is positioned over and fills the die cavity.

- Feed shoe retracts, scrapes away the excessive granulation, and levels the fill in the die cavity.

- Upper punch lowers and compresses the fill forming the tablet.

- Upper punch retracts as the lower punch rises with formed tablet to precise level of the stage.

- Feed shoe moves over the die cavity, shoves the tablet aside, and once again fills the cavity with granulation to repeat the process.

- Tablets fall into a collection container.

- Samples of tablets are assayed and tested for various quality standards.

- <u>Rotary tablet machines</u> equipped with <u>multiple punches and dies</u> operate via continuous rotating movement of punches.

- <u>A single rotary press with 16 stations</u> may produce <u>1150 tablets per minute</u>.

- <u>Double rotary tablet presses with 27,33,37,41,or 49 sets of punches and dies</u>

- Some of these machines can produce <u>10,000 or more tablets per minute</u> of operation.

- <u>Tablet dedusting</u>

- <u>To remove traces of loose powder adhering to tablets</u> following compression, tablets are conveyed directly from tableting machine to a deduster.

- <u>Compressed tablets</u> may then be <u>coated.</u>

- <u>Multiple-layer tablets</u> are produced by multiple feed and <u>multiple compression of fill material within a single die.</u>

- Tablets with an <u>inner core</u> are prepared by machines with special feed apparatus that places the core tablet precisely within the die for compression with surrounding fill.

- <u>Direct compression Tableting</u>

- Some granular chemicals, like <u>potassium chloride, possess</u> free flowing <u>and cohesive properties that enable them to be</u> compressed directly <u>in a tablet machine without need of granulation.</u>

- For chemicals lacking this quality, <u>special pharmaceutical excipients</u> may be used to impart necessary qualities for production of tablets by direct compression.

Fillers:

- Calcium salts—not used as fillers with tetracycline antibiotics-interaction

- Most preferred-lactose because of its solubility and compatibility

- MCC- easy compaction, compatibility and consistent uniformity of supply.

- **<u>FILLERS</u>**

- starch,

- powdered sucrose

- calcium phosphate

- **<u>Disintegrating agents</u>**

- croscarmellose,

- corn and potato starches,

- sodium starch glycolate,

- sodium carboxymethylcellulose,

- PVP, crosspovidone,

- cation exchange resins,

- alginic acid

- Croscarmellose(2%) and sodium starch glycolate (5%) preferred—because of their high water uptake and rapid action

- Starch- 5-10% is usually suitable.

- Upto 20% may be used to promote more rapid disintegration

- Often half is reserved and added to finished granulation prior to tablet formation

- Results in double disintegration of tablet

    One portion-breakup of tablet

    Other portion-assists in break up of pieces into fine particles

▫   Croscarmellose(2%) and sodium starch glycolate (5%) preferred—because of their high water uptake and rapid action

▪   Starch-   5-10% is usually suitable.

▫   Upto 20% may be used to promote more rapid disintegration

▪   Often half is reserved and added to finished granulation prior to tablet formation

▪   Results in double disintegration of tablet

>   One portion-breakup of tablet

>   Other portion-assists in break up of pieces into fine particles

▪   Preparing the damp mass

▪   Liquid binder is added to powder mixture-adhesion of powder particles.

▪   Dough is formed, used to prepare granulation

▪   Good binder-appropriate hardness and not hinder release of drug from tablet.

▫   Binding agents-povidone, an aq. Preparation of cornstarch (10-20%), glucose soln., (25-50%), molasses, methyl cellulose (3%), carboxymethyl cellulose and microcrystalline cellulose.

▪   If drug substance is adversely affected by an aqueous binder, a non- aqueous solution or dry binder may be used.

▪   Binding agent contributes to

▫   adhesion of granules and

▫   Maintains the integrity of tablet after compression.

▪   <u>Not overwet or underwet the powder</u>

▫   <u>Overwetting—result in granules that are too hard and</u>

▫   <u>Under wetting tablets--- that are too soft and tend to crumble</u>

▪   When desired a colorant or flavorant may be added to binding agent to prepare a granulation.

- Screening the damp mass into pellets or granules

  □ Wet mass pressed through screen (6 or 8 mesh) to prepare granules.

  □ May be done by hand or with special equipment.

  □ Spread evenly on large pieces of paper in shallow trays and dried.

Problems in tableting:

1 Capping

2 Lamination / Laminating

3 Chipping

4 Cracking

5 Sticking / Filming

6 Picking

7 Binding

8 Mottling

9 Double impression

- Capping, splitting, or laminating of tablets is sometimes related to air entrapment during direct compression.

- When air is trapped, resulting tablets expand when pressure of tableting is released, resulting in splits or layers in tablets.

- Capping, splitting:

- The top or bottom part of the tablet separates from the main body completely or partially.

- Laminating:

- The tablets breaks into two or more horizontal layers.

- Mottling:

- The unequal distribution of colors on the tablet surface.

- <u>Binding:</u>

- <u>Tablet adhere or tear in the die</u>

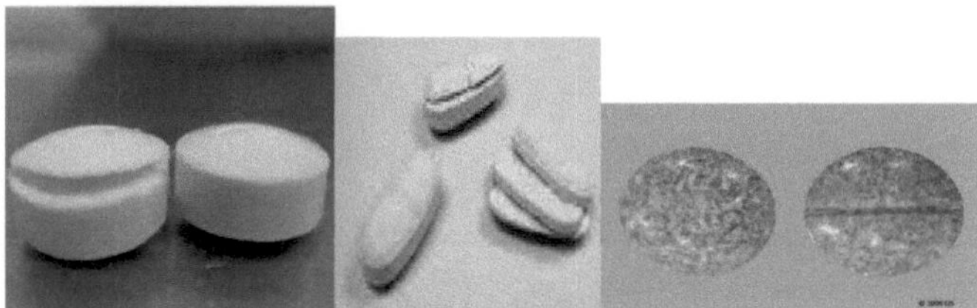

Picking

The materials gets off from the tablet surface and adhere to the face of the punches.

Sticking,

Adherence of granules to die walls

Chipping

Breaking of tablet edges.

- Capping also may be caused

by punches that are not immaculately clean and perfectly smooth or by a
, or fine powder.

▫ Fine powder, which results when a dried granulation is sized, is generally <u>10-20% of weight of granulation.</u>

- Some fine is desired to fill the die cavity properly.

- Excess can lead to tablet softness and capping.

- Tablets that have aged or been stored improperly also may exhibit <u>splitting or other physical deformations.</u>

- <u>References</u>

- 1. Allen, LV, Nicholas G, Ansel HC. Ansel's Pharmaceutical Dosage Forms and Drug Delivery Systems (9th ed.), Lippincott Williams & Wilkins, 2011(Latest edition).

- 2. Sinko PJ. Martin's Physical Pharmacy and Pharmaceutical Sciences (6th ed.), Lippincott Williams & Wilkins; 2010(Latest edition)

- 3. Aulton, M.E. Pharmaceutics: The Science of dosage form design, (2nd ed.), Churchill Livingstone, (Latest edition).

Chapter 5.

TABLET COATING TECHNIQUES

Objectives

1. To know Tablet Coating concepts

2. To understand the History of coating,

3. To explain Supercell Coating process

4. To kow and explain Magnetically Assisted Impaction Coating process

INTRODUCTION

Tablet is a pharmaceutical solid dosage form, comprising a mixture of active substances and excipients, usually in powder form, pressed or compacted into a solid. Tablets Dosage form is one of a most preferred dosage form all over the world. Almost all drug molecules can be formulated in a tablet and process of manufacturing of tablets is very simple, and is very flexible. Coating is a process by which an essentially dry, outer layer of coating material is applied to the surface of a dosage form to achieve specific benefits. Coating may be applied to a wide range of oral solid dosage form, including tablets, capsules, multiparticulates and drug crystals. When coating composition is applied to a batch of tablets in a coating pan, the tablet surfaces become covered with a tacky polymeric film. Before the tablet surface dries, the applied coating changes from a sticky liquid to tacky semisolid and eventually to a nonsticky dry surface pans1. Many solid pharmaceutical dosage forms are produced with coatings, either on the external surface of the tablet, or on materials dispensed within gelatine capsules. The tablet should release the medicament gradually and the drug should be available for digestion. The coating process can be specially formulated to regulate how fast the tablet dissolves and where the active drugs are to be absorbed into the body after ingestion2.

PRIMARY COMPONENTS INVOLVED IN TABLET COATING

1)Tablet properties

2)Coating process, design and control Coating equipments

Parameters of the coating process Facility and ancillary equipments Automation in coating processes. Tablet Properties

Tablets that are to be coated must possess some proper physical characteristics. The tablets roll in a coating pan. To tolerate the intense attrition of tablets striking other tablets orwalls of the coating equipment, the tablets must be resistant to abrasion and chipping.

Coating Process, Design & Control

In most coating methods, the coating solutions are sprayed onto the tablets as the tablets are being agitated in a pan, fluid bed, etc. As the solution is being sprayed, a thin film is formed that adheres directly to each tablet. The coating may be formed by a single application or may be built up in layers through the use of multiple spraying cycles. Rotating coating pans are often used in the pharmaceutical industry. Uncoated tablets are placed in the pan and the liquid coating solution is introduced into the pan while the tablets are tumbling. The liquid portion of the coating solution is then evaporated by passing air over the surface of the tumbling tablets. In contrast, a fluid bed coater operates by passing air through a bed of tablets at a velocity sufficient to support and separate the tablets as individual units. Once separated, the tablets are sprayed with the coating composition. The coating process is usually consisting of the following steps:

a. Batch identification and Recipe selection (film or sugar coating)

b. Loading/Dispensing (accurate dosing of all required raw materials)

c. Warming

d. Spraying (application and rolling are carried out simultaneously)

e. Drying

f. Cooling

g. Unloading

Coating Equipment

A modern tablet coating system combines several components:

a. A coating pan

b. A spraying system

c. An air handling unit

d. A dust collector

Benefits of Tablet Coating

Tablets coating mask the taste, odour, or colour of the drug. Tablets coating control the release of the drug from the tablet. It provides physical and chemical protection and protects the drug from the gastric environment of the stomach (acid resistant enteric coating). Incorporate of another drug or formula adjuvant in the coating to avoid chemical incompatibilities or to provide sequential drug release, improvement of pharmaceutical elegance by use of special colours and contrasting printing can also be obtained from tablet coating.

Shortcomings of Tablet Coating

Sugar coating carries relatively high cost, long coating time and high bulk due to the use of other coating materials. It is tedious, time-consuming and requires the expertise of highly skilled technician.

HISTORY OF COATING TECHNIQUE

"Panning" was the original word for the process of adding a coating to a tablet. The word panning is still a common term which is used in the confectionary business. In past years coating perform basically using a rotating drum (pan) on a stand. A coating solution was added, while the rotation of the pan distributed the solution throughout the bed of tablets. The main disadvantage of this technology was slow waiting for the coating solution to dry; and the trick was to get it to dry evenly. With the advent of film coating a film or thin membrane, usually representing 1-3% of the total tablet weight, was sprayed on using a perforated pan. To decrease the overall process time, holes were made through the pan so that treated air (hot or cold) could be pulled through the pan, much like a clothes dryer, allowing the tablets to dry more quickly. With this advent of improved drying came the ability to switch the film coating solution from a solvent based solution to a water based solution.

Coating of pharmaceutical dosage forms has been practiced for many centuries. The historical development of coating technique is mentioned below:-

LAST 40 YEARS:-

Features

• Introduction of the side- vented tablet coating pans (with perforations), Figure 1,

• Evolution was required for the introduction of aqueous based film coating polymers to the pharmaceutical industry

• Carbon steel construction except for pan

• Many screws, not welded in places

• Does not complies GMP

LAST 30 YEARS:-

Introduction of reliable microprocessor based process control systems required to insure process control and repeatability. Features

• Improved design spray nozzles for tablet coating

• specific applications (all stainless steel)

• Improved air preparation systems required for consistent aqueous process drying

• Improved GMP coater design, more cleanable, all stainless steel (Figure 2)

• Improved tablet handling

• All required for the optimization of aqueous film coating process

LAST 20 YEARS:-

Features

• Potable water storage tank.

• Washing nozzles (coater mounted).

• Reduced cleaning time

• Cleaning of the areas, that are difficult to access

• Conservation of cleaning solution

• Standardization of the cleaning process

- Energy conservation

LAST 10 YEARS

• More advanced film coating spray nozzles with anti- bearding designs

• More reliable industrial automation for accurate and repeatable control of process parameters ie: dewpoint, mass solution flow, air flow etc.

• The evolution of the improvements to the batch tablet coater has allowed the recent advancements in continuous tablet coating

TRADITIONAL COATING TECHNIQUES:-

Generally three methods are used for tablet coating

1. SUGAR COATING

2. FILM COATING

3. ENTERIC COATING SUGAR COATING:-

Sugar coating process involves five separate operations:

I. Sealing/Water proofing: provides a moisture barrier and harden the tablet surface.

II.   Subcoating causes a rapid buildup the tablet size and to round off the tablet edges.

III.   Grossing/Smoothing: smoothes out the subcoated surface and increases the tablet size to predetermine dimension.

IV.   Colouring gives the tablet its color and finished size.

V.   Polishing produces the characteristics gloss.

The characteristics of sugar coating technique has been given below (Table 1)

Table No. 1:- Characteristic of Sugar Coating

Type	CHARACTERISTIC	SUGAR COATING
Tablet	Appearance	Rounded with high degree of polish
	Weight increase because of coating material	30-50%
	Logo or 'break lines'	Not possible
Process	Operator training required	Considerable
	Adaptability to GMP	Difficulty may arise
	Process stages	Multistage process
	Functional coatings	Not usually possible apart from enteric coating[6]

Table No. 2: Materials Used in Film Coating

S. No.	Material	Type	Uses	Examples
1.	Film Former	Enteric Non Enteric	To control the release of drug	Hydroxy Propyl Methyl Cellulose (HPMC), Methyl Hydroxy Ethyl Cellulose (MHEC)
2.	Solvents		To dissolve or disperse the polymers	IPA and Methylene chloride
3.	Plasticizer	Internal Plasticizing External Plasticizi	It Pertains to the chemical modification of the basic polymer that alters the physical properties of the polymer. It incorporated with	Glycerol, Propylene glycol, PEG 200-6000 Grades Diethyl phthalate (DEP), Dibutyl phthalate (DBP) and Tributyl citrate (TBC)

			the primary polymeric film former, changes the flexibility, tensile strength, or adhesion properties of the resulting film	
4.	Colourants	Inorganic materials Natural coloring materials	For light shade: concentration of less than 0.01% may be used For dark shade: concentration of more than 2.0% may be required.	Iron Oxides Anthocyanins, Caramel, Carotenoids,
5.	Opaquant-Extenders	----------	Formulations to provide more pastel colours and increase film coverage	Titanium dioxide, silicate (talc &aluminum silicates), carbonates(magnesium carbonates) 3

Table No. 3:- Characteristic of Film Coating

Type	CHARACTERISTIC	FILM COATING
Tablet	Appearance	Retain contour of original core. Usually not as shiny as sugar coat type
	Weight increase because of coating material	2-3%
	Logo or 'break lines'	Possible
Process	Operator training required	Process tends itself to automation and easy training of operator
	Adaptability to GMP	High
	Process stages	Usually single stage

| Functional coatings | Easily adaptable for controlled release[6] |

FILM COATING:-

Development of Film Coating Formulations:-

If the following questions are answered concomitantly then one can go for film coating:

i) Is it necessary to mask objectionable taste, color and odor?

ii)Is it necessary to control drug release?

iii)   What tablets size, shape, or color constrains must be placed on the developmental work?

Ideal requirements of film coating materials:

i) Solubility in solvent of choice for coating preparation

ii)Solubility requirement for the intended use e.g. free water-solubility, slow water solubility or pH -dependent solubility

iii)   Capacity to produce an elegant looking product

iv)   High stability against heat, light, moisture, air and the substrate being coated

v)   No inherent colour, taste or odor

vi)   High compatibility with other coating solution additives

vii)   Nontoxic with no pharmacological activity

viii)   High resistance to cracking

ix)   Film former should not give bridging or filling of the debossed tablet

x)Compatible to printing procedure

There are various materials used in film coating as shown in table no. 2. Table no. 3 summarizes the characteristics of film coating.

ENTERIC COATING:-

• Ideal Properties of Enteric Coating Materials:-

- Resistance to gastric fluids.

- Susceptible/permeable to intestinal fluid.

- Compatibility with most coating solution components and the drug substrate.

- Formation of continuous film.

- Nontoxic, cheap and ease of application.

- Ability to be readily printed.

Polymers Used For Enteric Coating Are As Follow:-

1. Cellulose acetate phthalate (CAP)

2. Acrylate polymers

3. Hydroxy propyl methyl cellulose phthalate

4. Polyvinyl acetate phthalate3, 19

RECENT TRENDS IN TABLET COATING TECHNIQUES:-

ELECTROSTATIC DRY COATING:

An electrostatic dry powder coating process for tablets was developed for the first time by electrostatic dry powder coating in a pan coater system .The optimized dry powder coating process produces tablets with smooth surface, good coating uniformity and release profile that are comparable to that of the tablet cores. This novel electrostatic dry powder coating technique is an alternative to aqueous or solvent based coating process for pharmaceutical products

The electrostatic coating process is widely useful in food technology, paint technology, metal coatings, coating of living cells and coating of tablets as well as capsules. The principle of electrostatic powder coating states that spraying of a mixture of finely grounded particles and polymers onto a substrate surface without using any solvent and then heating the substrate for curing on oven until the powder mixture is fused into film (Figure 6)

Figure 6: Schematic diagram of electrostatic dry coating.

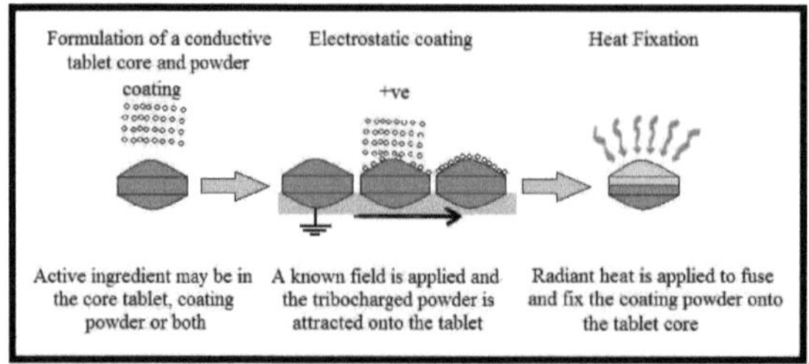

According to the charging mechanism, there are two types of spraying units:

a) Corona charging

b) Tribo charging.

Mechanism of Corona charging:

In this mechanism, the electrical breakdown and ionization of air by imposing high voltage on a sharp pointed needle like electrode (i.e. charging pin) at the outlet of the gun. The powder particles pick up the negative ions on their way from the gun to the substrate. The movement of particles between the substrate and the charging gun is done by the combination of electrical and mechanical forces. The mechanical forces generated by the air blows the powder towards the substrate from the spray gun. The electrical forces are derived from the electrical field between the earthen substance and the charging tip of the spray gun, and from the repulsive forces between the charged particles. The electrical field can be adjusted to direct the powder's flow, control pattern size, shape, and powder density as it is released from the gun.

Mechanism of tribo charging:

In the tribo charging, it makes the use of the principle of friction charging associated with the dielectric properties of solid materials and so that no free ions and electrical field will be present between the spray gun and grounded substance. For tribo charging guns, the electrical forces are only regarded to the repulsive forces between the charged particles. After spraying, charged particles come into the space adjacent to the substrate and the attraction forces between the grounded substrate and the charged particles makes the particle to deposit on the substrate. Chargedparticles are sprayed uniformly onto the earthen substrate in virtue of mechanical forces and electrostatic attraction. Particles deposit on the substrate before the repulsion force of the deposited particles against the coming particles increase and exceed the electrostatic attraction. Finally once the repulsion force becomes equivalent to the attraction force, particles cannot adhere to the substrate any more, and the coating thickness does not increase any more. Electrostatic dry coating of electrically non-conducting substrates and pharmaceutical tablet cores is more difficult. For secure the coating to the core, the powder must be transformed into a film without damaging the tablet core, which usually includes organic materials. In addition, an even coating is required and it is difficult to obtain an even coating of powder on a tablet core. Various properties of powder such as particle size distribution, chemical composition, tribo and corona charging characteristics, electrical resistivity, hygroscopicity, fluidity and shape distribution play significant role on the performance of powder coating such as transfer efficiency, film thickness, adhesion and appearance. Distance, nozzle geometry, and composition of the precursor solution play an important role in the electrostatic coating process.

MAGNETICALLY ASSISTED IMPACTION COATING (MAIC):

A Technique is developed for estimating the coating time in a magnetically assisted impaction coating (MAIC) device. The mixture of the host, guest and magnetic particles is assumed to stay in a fluidized state where the distribution of velocities is a Maxwell–Boltzman type. It is assumed that the collisions occurs among the particles are important for impinging the guest particles onto the surface of host particles, and thus forming a semi-permanent coating on the surface of host particles. The coating time is depend on several parameters, including the number density of host particles, the diameter ratio of the host and guest particles, the height of the fluidized particle bed and the material properties of the host and guest particles. There is an optimal value of the bed height for which the coating time is a minimum. The coating

time increases sharply when the bed height is smaller or larger than the optimal value, and also when the diameter of host particles is increased.

Various dry coating methods have been developed such as compression coating, plasticizer dry coating, heat dry coating and electrostatic dry coating. These methods generally allow for the application of high shearing stresses or high impaction forces or exposure to higher temperature for coating. The strong mechanical forces and the accompanying heat generated can cause layering and even embedding of the guest particles onto the surface of the host particles. Many foods and pharmaceutical ingredients, being organic and relatively very soft, are very sensitive to heat and can quite easily be deformed by severe mechanical forces. Hence, some soft coating methods that can attach the guest (coating material) particles onto the host (material to be coated) particles with a minimum degradation of particle size, shape and composition caused by the build up of heat are the best candidates for such applications. The magnetically assisted impaction coating (MAIC) devices can coat soft organic host and guest particles without changing in the material shape and size. Although there is some heat generated on a minute level due to the collisions of particles during MAIC, but it is negligible. This is an additional advantage when dealing with temperature sensitive powders such as pharmaceuticals.

Magnetically Assisted Impaction Coating (MAIC) is being developed to improve the effectiveness of mixing powders with nano-sized particles without the aid of a solvent or heat. In general, uniform mixing of nano-sized materials is more difficult than mixing of larger sized materials. Still in development, the technology will aid manufacturing applications in producing higher quality products.

Mechanism of coating in the MAIC process:

There are few stages in the mechanism of coating of MAIC process is

Stage-I: Excitation of magnetic particles.

Stage-II: De-agglomeration of guest particles (coating material).

Stage-III: Shearing and spreading of guest particles on the surface of the host particles (material to be coated).

Stage-IV: Magnetic-host-host particle interaction. Stage-V: Magnetic–host–wall interaction and Stage-VI: Formation of coated products.

AQUEOUS FILM COATING TECHNOLOGY

The sugar coating process is very time consuming and it is depending on the skills of coating operator, this technique has been replaced by film coating technology. This technique was started with the use of organic solvents like methylene chloride but now has been replaced with aqueous film coating due to environmental and regulatory considerations. Moreover the cost of any organic solvent is far more than the cost of purified water. Therefore, the conversion from organic solvent based coating to aqueous solvent based coating makes the coating process more economical, though initially it may need a little more investment to upgrade the coating facility. The need of this upgradation arises due to the need of higher drying capacity (the latent heat of water is 2200 kJ as compared to 550 kJ for methylene chloride which implies that to evaporate water one will need 4 times more energy as compared to methylene chloride)12. The figure of enteric aqueous film coating tablets has been shown in figure 8.

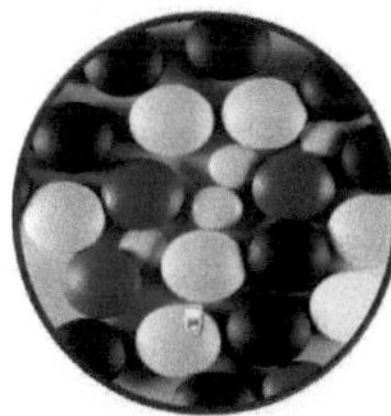

Figure 8:- Enteric aqueous film coating tablets

The problems associated with organic solvent-based film coating and the advantages of aqueous based systems have long been recognized. Film coating technology has now advanced to the level where aqueous coating has become a matter of routine coating rather than the exception. The successful introduction of a wide variety of aqueous based film coating products (by M/s. Ideal Cures Pvt. Ltd., under the brand name INSTACOAT) has resulted in easy conversion from organic solvent based coatings to aqueous film coating for several companies; many of them still use the conventional coating equipment.

Development of film coating formulation

The optimization of film coating formulation may be necessary to improve adhesion of the coating to the core material, to decrease bridging of intagliations, to increase coating hardness or to improve any other property that the formulator deems deficient. The development scientist has to consider three major factors which can affect the film quality- tensile strength of the film coating formulation (mainly dependant on polymer properties), elasticity of the resultant film (mainly dependant on properties and quantity of plasticizer used) and the film-tablet surface interaction (each and every ingredient used in the coating formulation can affect this interaction and can change the adhesion properties of the film on the tablet surface). Due to these important factors, it becomes very important to use the most optimized coating formulations in order to get the best results.

SUPERCELL COATING TECHNOLOGY:-

Supercell Coating Technology is a revolutionary tablet coating that accurately deposits controlled amounts of coating materials on tablets—even if they are extremely hygroscopic or friable. Inconsistent and simperfect condition, this "standard" practice of tablet coating often delivers a non- homogenous product. Because the tablets are loaded in large rotating pans and vented for hot air drying, edges of tablets can get grounded off, intagliations can get filled in by coating material, and edges and corners may not be coated with the same thickness as the tablet faces. The inaccuracy in deposition of coating material limits the use of modified release coatings (figure 9). In a laboratory, it is necessary to coat several kilograms of tablets at one time, making R&D of a tablet dosage form costly and difficult.

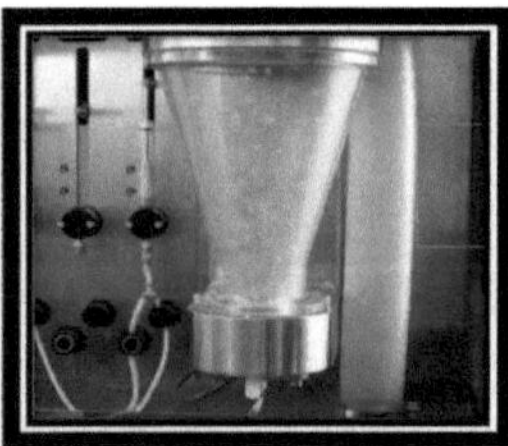

Figure 9:- Supercell Coating Technology

Furthermore, extremely hygroscopic tablets cannot be coated with current technology, nor can flat or other odd shapes be consistently coated. This process must be run slowly to prevent "twinning," where two or more tablets stick together. Tablets may also be coated in a Wurster-type coating apparatus, but tablet attrition generally prevents all but the hardest tablets from being coated this way.

TABLET COATING DEFECTS

An ideal tablet should be free from any visual defect or functional defect. The advancements and innovations in tablet manufacture have not decreased the problems, often encountered in the production, instead have increased the problems, mainly because of the complexities of tablet presses; and/or the greater demands of quality. An industrial pharmacist usually encounters number of problems during manufacturing. Majority of visual defects are due to inadequate fines or inadequate moisture in the granules ready for compression or due to faulty machine setting. Functional defects are due to faulty formulation. Solving many of the manufacturing problems requires an in-depth knowledge of granulation processing and tablet presses, and is acquired only through an exhaustive study and a rich experience17,18,25. Here, we will discuss the imperfections found in tablets along-with their causes and related remedies (see table no. 5). Several tablets are being shown in figure no. 11.The imperfections are known as: 'VISUAL DEFECTS' and they are either related to imperfections in anyone or more of the following factors:

Table No. 5: Tablet Coating Defects with Reason and Their Remedies

S. No.	Tablet defects	Definition	Reason	Remedies
1.	Blistering	It is local detachment of film from the substrate forming blister.	Entrapment of gases in the film due to overheating either during spraying or at the end of the coating run.	Milder drying conditions are warranted in this case.
2.	Chipping	It is defect where the film becomes chipped and dented, usually at the edges of the tablet.	Decrease in fluidizing air or speed of rotation of the drum in pan coating	Be careful not to over-dry the tablets in the preheating stage. That can make the tablets brittle and promote capping.
3.	Picking	It is defect where isolated areas of film are pulled away from the surface when the	Conditions similar to cratering that produces an overly wet tablet bed where adjacent tablets can	A reduction in the liquid application rate or increase in the drying air temperature and air volume usually solves this problem.

		tablet sticks together and then part.	stick together and then break apart.	Excessive tackiness may be an indication of a poor formulation.
4.	Twin ning	This is the term for two tablets that stick together	Common problem with capsule shaped tablets.	Assuming you don't wish to change the tablet shape, you can solve this problem by balancing the pan speed and spray rate. Try reducing the spray rate or increasing the pan speed. In some cases, it is necessary to modify the design of the tooling by very slightly changing the radius. The change is almost impossible to see, but it prevents the twinning problem.
5.	Pittin g	It is defect whereby pits occur in the surface of a tablet core without any visible disruption of the film coating.	Temperature of the tablet core is greater than the melting point of the materials used in the tablet formulation.	Control the temperature of tablet core during the formulation
6.	Crate ring	It is defect of film coating whereby volcanic-like craters appears exposing the tablet surface.	The coating solution penetrates the surface of the tablet, often at the crown where the surface is more porous, causing localized disintegration of the core and disruption of the coating.	---------------
7.	Bloo ming	It is defect where coating becomes dull immediately or after prolonged storage at high temperatures.	It is due to collection on the surface of low molecular weight ingredients included in the coating formulation. In most circumstances the ingredient will be plasticizer.	---------------
8.	Blush ing	It is defect best described as	It is thought to be due to precipitated	

		whitish specks or haziness in the film.	polymer exacerbated by the use of high coating temperature at or above the thermal gelation temperature of the polymers.	---------------
9.	Colo ur variat ion	A defect which involves variation in colour of the film.	Alteration of the frequency and duration of appearance of tablets in the spray zone or the size/shape of the spray zone.	A reformulation with different plasticizers and additives is the best way to solve film instabilities caused by the ingredients
10.	Crack ing or Splitt ing	It is defect in which the film either cracks across the crown of the tablet (cracking) or splits around the edges of the tablet (Splitting)	Internal stress in the film exceeds tensile strength of the film.	tensile strength of the film can be increased by Using higher molecular weight polymers or polymer blends
11.	Infilli ng	It is defect that renders the intagliations indistinctness.	Inability of foam, formed by air spraying of a polymer solution, to break. The foam droplets on the surface of the tablet breakdown readily due to attrition but the intagliations form a protected area allowing the foam to accumulate and "set". Once the foam has accumulated to a level approaching the outer contour of the tablet surface, normal attrition ca n occur allowing the	Judicious monitoring of the fluid application rate and thorough mixing of the tablets in the pan can prevent filling.

| 12. | Oran
ge
peel/
Roug
hness | It is surface defect resulting in the film being rough and nonglossy. Appearance is similar to that of an orange. | Inadequate spreading of the coating solution before drying. | 1. Thinning the solution with additional solvent may correct this problem.

2. Moving the nozzle closer to the tablet bed and reducing the degree of atomization can decrease the roughness due to "spray drying". |
| 13. | Mottl
ing | Mottling is uneven distribution of the colour on the surface of the tablet, with dark and light patches on it. | It is mainly due to different colouration of the excipient or the degradation product of the tablet is coloured. | Coating solution prepare properly in sufficient quantity. |

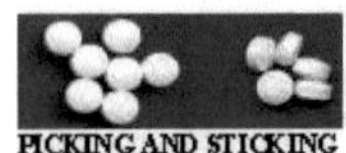

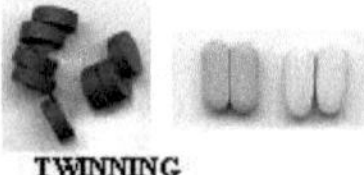

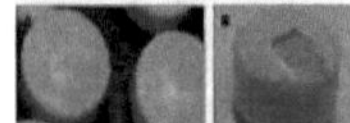

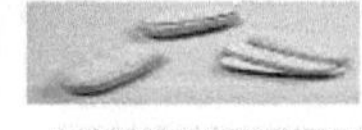

References:

1. 1. Gupta Ankit et al. IRJP 2012, 3 (9)

2. Allen, LV, Nicholas G, Ansel HC. Ansel's Pharmaceutical Dosage Forms and Drug Delivery Systems (9th ed.), Lippincott Williams & Wilkins, 2011(Latest edition).

3. Sinko PJ. Martin's Physical Pharmacy and Pharmaceutical Sciences (6th ed.), Lippincott Williams & Wilkins; 2010(Latest edition)

4. Aulton, M.E. Pharmaceutics: The Science of dosage form design, (2nd ed.), Churchill Livingstone, (Latest edition).

CHAPTER.6

Evaluation of Pharmaceutical Tablets

Objectives:

1. To describe pharmaceutical tablets dosage form.

2. To evaluate Pharmaceutical tablets testing: weight variation test, Tablet hardness test, Tablet Friability test, Tablet disintegration test, Dissolution test

3. To perform pharmaceutical calculation.

4. To Interpret results.

Pharmaceutical tablets dosage form.

Tablets are solid preparations each containing a single dose of one or more active ingredients. They are normally prepared by compression although some tablets are prepared by moulding.

Many different types of tablets are available, which may be in a variety of shapes and sizes. These include dispersible or effervescent, chewable, sublingual and buccal tablets, lozenges, tablets for vaginal administration and solution tablets. Some tablets are designed to release the medication slowly for prolonged drug release and sustained drug action.

In addition to the active ingredient, several excipients, or inactive ingredients are added.. These aid the process of tableting and ensure that the active ingredients are released in the body as intended. Excipients include:

1. Diluents or fillers: These add bulk to make the tablet easier to handle. Examples include lactose, mannitol, microcrystalline cellulose and calcium carbonate.

2. Binders or adhesives: These enable granules to be prepared which improve flow properties of the mixture and compression. Examples include acacia, mucilage, glucose, povidone and starch mucilage.

3. Disintegrators or disintegrating agents. These ensure that the tablet breaks down into its component particles after ingestion. Examples include sodium alginate, carmellose sodium, microcrystalline cellulose, sodium glycin carbonate and starch.

4. Antiadherents, glidants, lubricants or lubricating agents:

-Lubricants are essential for flow of the tablet material into the tablet dies and preventing sticking of the compressed tablet in the punch and die. Examples of lubricants are magnesium and calcium stearate, sodium lauryl sulphate and sodium stearyl fumarate.

-Colloidal silica is usually the glidant of choice.

-Talc and magnesium stearate are effective antiadherents.

5. Miscellaneous agents may be added, such as colours and flavours in chewable tablets.

❖   Some tablets have coatings, such as sugar coating or film coating. Coating can protect the tablet from environmental damage, mask an unpleasant flavour, aid identification of the tablet and enhance its appearance. Enteric coatings on tablets resist dissolution or disruption of the tablet in the stomach, but not in the intestine. This is useful when a drug is destroyed by gastric acid, is irritating to the gastric mucosa, or when by passing the stomach aids drug absorption.

➢   **Shelf life and storage**

Shelf life specifies the period of time which a product can be stored, under specified conditions, and remain in optimum condition and suitable for consumption.

The shelf life of a drug is loosely defined here as the length of time a drug can stay on the shelf without degrading to unacceptable levels.

Most tablets should be stored in air – tight packaging, protected from light and extremes of temperature. When stored properly they generally have a long shelf life. Some tablets need to be stored in a cool place, for example, Ketovite (store between 2 and 8 ^{0}C) and Leukeran (chlorambucil) (store under 15 ^{0}C).

Some tablets contain volatile drugs, for example glyceryl trinitrate, and must be packed in glass containers with tightly fitting metal screw caps. An additional warning must be placed on the tablets, when dispensed to patients, to advise them to throw away the tablets 8 weeks after opening, as they lose potency.

➢ **Containers**

Strip or blister packs are dispensed in a paperboard box and tablets counted from bulk containers are placed in amber glass or plastic containers with airtight, child- resistant closures.

Pharmaceutical tablets testing: weight variation test, Tablet hardness test, Tablet Friability test , Tablet disintegration test.

➢ **Quality Standards and compendial requirements**

In addition to the apparent features of tablets, tablets must meet physical specifications and quality standards. These include criteria for weight, weight variation, content uniformity, thickness, hardness, disintegration, and dissolution. These factors ensure that established product quality standards are met.

1)   Tablet weight and USP weight variation test

The quantity of fill in the die of a tablet press determines the weight of the tablet. The volume of fill is adjusted with the first few tablets to yield the desired weight and content. The USP contains a test for determination of dosage for determination of dosage form uniformity by weight variation for uncoated tablets. In the test,

- 10 tablets are dusted and weighed individually using the analytical balance

- The average weight and standard deviation are calculated.

- According to the USP, the requirements for uniformity are met if each individual tablet is within 85% to 115% of the mean.

The individual tablet weights are then compared to the average weight. Not more than two of the tablets must differ from the average weight by not more than the percentages stated in Table 1.

The USP has provided limits for the average weight of uncoated compressed tablets.

Table 1: Weight variation requirements

Average weight	Percent difference
130mg or less	10
More than 130mg through 324mg	7.5
More than 324mg	5

2)   Content uniformity

By the USP method 10 dosage units are individually assayed for their content according to the method described in the individual monograph. Unless otherwise stated in the monograph, the requirements for content uniformity are met if the amount of active ingredient in each dosage unit lies within the range of 85% to 115% of the label claim and the standard deviation is less than 6%. If one or more dosage units do not meet these criteria, additional tests as prescribed in the USP are required.

3)   Tablet thickness

The thickness of a tablet is determined by the diameter of the die, the amount of fill permitted to enter the die, the compaction characteristics of the fill material, and the force or pressure applied during compression.

To produce tablets of uniform thickness during and between batch productions for the same formulation, care must be exercised to employ the same factors of fill, die, and pressure. The degree of pressure affects not only thickness but also hardness of the tablet; hardness is perhaps the more important criterion, since it can affect disintegration and dissolution. Thus, for tablets of uniform thickness and hardness, it is doubly important to control pressure. Tablet thickness may be measured by hand gauge during production or by automated equipment.

- Ten tablets are dusted and using forceps are individually placed between the calipers of the thickness tester

- The instrument gives a visual reading of tablet thickness.

4)   Tablet hardness

Hardness determines the crushing strength of the tablets. Generally, the greater the pressure applied, the harder the tablets, although the characteristics of the granulation also have a bearing on hardness. Certain tablets, such as lozenges and buccal tablets, that are intended to dissolve slowly, intentionally are made hard; other tablets, such as those for immediate drug release, are made soft. In general, tablets should be sufficiently hard to resist breaking during normal handling and yet soft enough to disintegrate properly after swallowing.

Special dedicated hardness testers or multifunctional systems are used to measure the degree of force (in kilograms, pounds, or in arbitrary units) required to break a tablet. A force of about 4-6 kg is considered the minimum requirement for a satisfactory tablet. Multifunctional automated equipment can determine weight, hardness, thickness, and diameter of the tablet.

- Using forceps, 10 tablets are individually placed between the platens of the hardness tester

- The test button is pushed and the instrument gives a visual reading of tablet hardness

5)   Tablet Friability

It is USP test to determine how well tablets will stand up to coating, packaging, shipping, and other processing conditions. A tablet's durability may be determined through the use of a friabilator. This apparatus determines the tablet's friability, or tendency to crumble, by allowing it to roll and fall within the drum.

- Ten tablets are dusted and weighed on the analytical balance

- The tablets are placed in the section 1 of the drum of the friability tester and rotated 100 times

- The tablets are re-dusted and re-weighed and any loss in weight is noted.

- Resistance to loss of weight indicates the tablets ability to withstand abrasion in handling, packaging, and shipment. A maximum weight loss of not more than 1% generally is considered acceptable for most products.

6) Tablet disintegration

For the medicinal agent in a tablet to become fully available for absorption, the tablet must first disintegrate and discharge the drug to the body fluids for dissolution. Tablet disintegration also is important for tablets containing medicinal agents (such as antacids and antidiarrheals) that are not intended to be absorbed but rather to act locally within the gastrointestinal tract. In these instances, tablet disintegration provides drug particles with an increased surface area for activity within the gastrointestinal tract.

All USP tablets must pass a test for disintegration, which is conducted in vitro using a testing apparatus. The apparatus consists of a basket and rack assembly containing six open-ended transparent tubes of USP-specified dimensions, held vertically upon a 10-mesh stainless steel wire screen. During testing, a tablet is placed in each of the six tubes of the basket, and through the use of a mechanical device, the basket is raised and lowered in the immersion fluid at 29 to 32 cycles per minute, the wire screen always below the level of the fluid. For uncoated tablets, buccal tablets, and sublingual tablets, water at about 37^0C serves as the immersion fluid unless another fluid is specified in the individual monograph. For these tests, complete disintegration is defined as "that state in which any residue of the unit, except fragments of insoluble coating or capsule shell, remaining on the screen of the test apparatus is a soft mass having no palpably firm core".

Tablets must disintegrate within the times set forth in the individual monograph, usually 30 minutes, but varying from about 2 minutes for nitroglycerin tablets to up to 4 hours for buccal tablets.

If one or more tablets fail to disintegrate, additional tests prescribed by the USP must performed.

Enteric-coated tablets are similarly tested, except that the tablets are tested in simulated gastric fluid for 1 hour, after which no sign of disintegration, cracking, or softening must be seen. They are then actively immersed in the simulated intestinal fluid for the time stated in the individual monograph, during which time the tablets disintegrate completely for a positive test.

USP test to determine the time required for tablets to disintegrate

- A 900 ml beaker is filled with water and maintained at 37 ± 2^0 C.

- Six tablets are placed into the basket-rack assembly and connected to the disintegration apparatus

- The apparatus and the timer are started simultaneously and the time required for the last tablet to disintegrate is recorded.

Method of calculation and Interpretation of results.

Example on weight variation test:

In assaying the drug content of a sample of tablets, the following values were obtained:-

Weight   Weight Table 1: Weight variation requirements

(g)   (mg)

0.628g = 628mg

0.607g = 607mg

0.622g = 622mg

0.627g = 627mg

0.622g = 622mg

0.621g = 621mg

0.623g = 623mg

0.625g = 625mg

0.619g = 619mg

0.624g = 624mg

Average weight	Percent difference
130mg or less	10
More than 130mg through 324mg	7.5
More than 324mg	5

6218mg

$$\text{Mean} = \frac{\text{Sum of values}}{\text{Number of values}} = \frac{6218}{10} = 621.8 \quad (5 \times 621.8)/100 = 31.09$$

5% = 31.09

621.8 + 31.1 = 652.89

621.8 – 31.1 = 590.70

Standard Deviation

In assaying the drug content of a sample of tablets, the following values were obtained:-

Weight (mg)	Deviation (mg)	(Deviation)^2
304	+4	16
295	-5	25
310	+10	100
305	+5	25
290	-10	100
306	+6	36
298	-2	4
293	-7	49
302	+2	4

297	-3	9
-------		-----------
3000		**368**

$$\textbf{Mean} = 3000/10 = 300\text{mg}, \quad \textbf{S.D.} = \sqrt{\frac{\sum d}{n-1}} = \sqrt{\frac{368}{9}} = \sqrt{40.9} = 6.4mg$$

<u>**Tablet Dissolution**</u>

- **In-vitro dissolution testing of solid dosage forms is important for a number of reasons**

1. **Guides formulation development toward product optimization.**

Dissolution studies in early stages of a product's development allow differentiation between formulations and correlations identified with in- vivo bioavailability data.

<u>**Microprocessor Programmable Digital Tablet Dissolution Test Apparatus**</u>

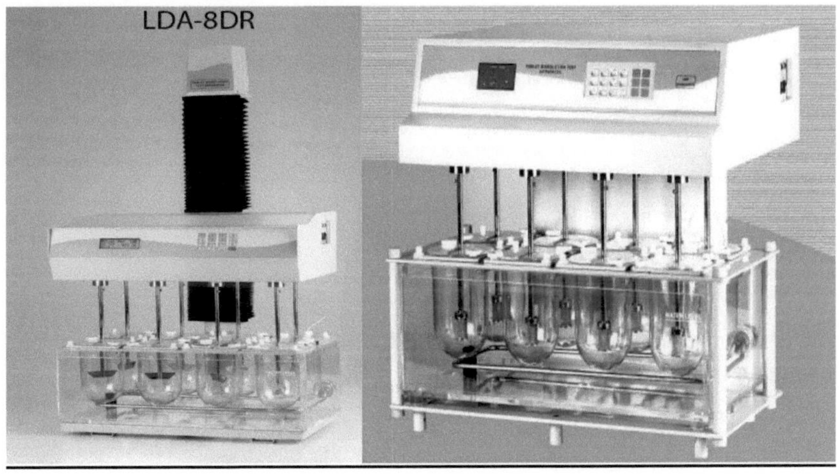

2. Manufacturing may be <u>monitored by dissolution testing</u> as a component of overall quality assurance program.

 Conduct of such testing from early product development through approval and commercial production ensures control of any variables of materials and processes that could affect dissolution and quality standards.

3. Consistent in-vitro dissolution testing ensures bioequivalence from batch to batch.

<u>It is a requirement for regulatory approval of marketing for products registered with the FDA and regulatory agencies of other countries</u>

- <u>Goal of in-vitro dissolution testing</u>

- Provide a reasonable prediction of or correlation with product's in-vivo bioavailability.

- System relates combinations of a drug's solubility (high or low) and its intestinal permeability (high or low) as basis for predicting the likelihood of achieving a successful invivo-invitro correlation.(1V1VC)

- High solubility and high permeability

- Low solubility and high permeability

- High solubility and low permeability

- low solubility and low permeability

For a high-solubility and high-permeability drug, an 1V1VC may be expected if dissolution rate is slower than the rate of gastric emptying In case of low-solubility and high-permeability drug, dissolution may be the rate-limiting step for absorption and 1V1VC may be expected.

In case of high solubility and low permeability, permeability is the rate –controlling step. and only limited 1V1VC may be possible.

- In case of a drug with low solubility and low permeability, significant problems are likely for oral drug delivery.

Tablet disintegration is the important first step to the dissolution

A number of formulation and manufacturing factors can affect disintegration and dissolution of tablet, including

- particle size of drug substance,
- solubility and hygroscopicity of formulation, type and conc. of disintegrant, binder, and lubricant,
- manufacturing method, particularly the compactness of granulation and compression force used in tableting

- USP includes seven apparatus designs for drug release and dissolution testing of

- Immediate-release oral dosage forms,

- Extended-release products,

- Enteric coated products and

- Transdermal drug delivery devices.

- USP Apparatus 1 and USP Apparatus 2-used principally for immediate-release solid oral dosage forms.

- Equipment consists of

- a) variable speed stirrer motor

- b) cylindrical stainless steel basket on stirrer shaft (USP apparatus 1)or a paddle as stirring element (USP apparatus 2)

- c) a 1000 ml vessel of glass or other inert transparent material fitted with a cover having centre port for the shaft of stirrer and three additional ports, two for removal of samples and one for a thermometer.

- d) a water bath to maintain the temperature of dissolution medium in the vessel.

- USP Apparatus 1—dosage unit is placed inside the basket.

- USP Apparatus 2—dosage unit is placed inside the vessel

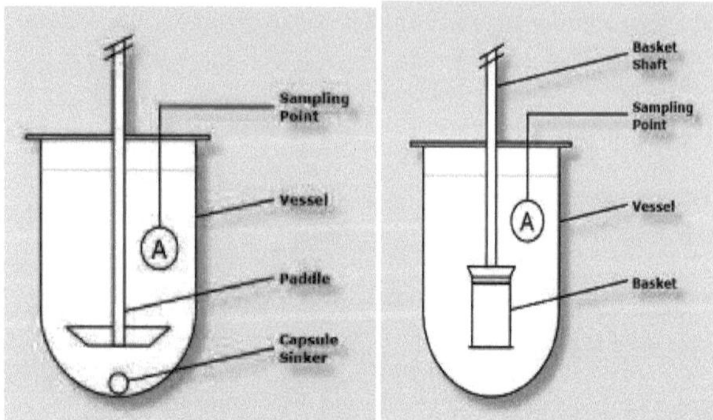

- In each test, vol. of dissolution medium is placed in the vessel and allowed to come to $37^0C + 0.5^0C$.

- Stirrer is rotated at the speed specified and at stated intervals, samples of medium are withdrawn for chemical analysis of proportion of drug dissolved.

- Tablet or capsule must meet the stated monograph requirement, for example, "not less than 85% of labeled amount is dissolved in 30 min".

- In-consistencies in dissolution occur not between dosage units from same batch but rather between batches or between products from different manufacturers.

- Pooled testing-----pooled specimens may be sampled from individual vessels or from multiple dosage units in a single vessel.

References

1.   Allen, LV, Nicholas G, Ansel HC. Ansel's Pharmaceutical Dosage Forms and Drug Delivery Systems (9th ed.), Lippincott Williams & Wilkins, 2011(Latest edition).

2.   Sinko PJ. Martin's Physical Pharmacy and Pharmaceutical Sciences (6th ed.), Lippincott Williams & Wilkins; 2010(Latest edition)

3.   Aulton, M.E. Pharmaceutics: The Science of dosage form design, (2nd ed.), Churchill Livingstone, (Latest edition).

Model-Questions

Definitions

1. Drug

An agent intended for use in the diagnosis, mitigation, treatment, cure, or   prevention of disease in humans or in other animals

2. Diagnosis

Process of identification of diseases

3. Mitigation

The action of reducing the severity,

4. Mydriatic drug

A mydriatic is an agent that induces dilation of the pupil.eg. Tropicamide

5. Miotic drug

Drug that causes miosis (constriction of the pupil of the eye) eg. pilocarpine

6. Diuretics

Diuretics are drugs that can increase the amount of water and sodium that is excreted in the urine.

Eg: Chlorothiazide

7. Expectorants

A medication that helps bring up mucus and other material from the lungs, bronchi, and trachea. Eg: Guaifenesin,

8. Cathartics

Cathartics increase the motility of the intestine or increase the bulk of feces. (Empties the bowel) EG: Bisacodyl

9. Laxatives

Mild Cathartics

EG: Polyethylene glycol

10. Analgesics

The term Analgesics encompasses a class of drugs that are designed to relieve pain without causing the loss of consciousness.

11. Glacoma

Glaucoma is a group of eye diseases causing optic nerve damage

12. Anesthetics

An anesthetic (or anaesthetic) is a drug that causes anesthesia, which is a reversible loss of sensation

13. Ebers papyrus

Most famous of surviving memorials is the Ebers papyrus a continuous scroll 60 feet long and a foot wide dating to the 16th century BC.

The text is dominated by drug formulas, with more than 800 formulas or prescriptions and more than 700 drugs mentioned.

14. Parenteral route

Located outside the alimentary canal. Taken into the body or administered in a manner other than through the digestive tract, as by intravenous or intramuscular injection.

15. Fillers

Substances added to increase the weight or size or fill space.

16. Thickeners

Substances added to increase the viscosity without modifying its other properties.

17. Suspending agent

Substances added to decrease the sedimentation of particles in suspension.

18. Disintegrants

Substances used to breakup of compacted mass in tablets or capsule.

19. Anti-microbial preservatives.

Substances added to protect from microbial growth.

Definitions:

Pharmacy-

Pharmacy is the science and technique of preparing as well as dispensing drugs and medicines

Pharmaceutics –

Pharmaceutics is the discipline of pharmacy that deals with the process of turning a new chemical entity (NCE) into a medication to be used safely and effectively

Diseases –

A disease is a particular abnormal, pathological condition that affects part or all of an organism

Fillers-

The substances used to increase the bulkiness of dosage form/ increase the weight of the dosage form

- Thickeners - The substances used to increase the viscosity of dosage form

- Solvents – The substances used to dissolve the drug particles.

- Suspending agents – The substances used to suspend the insoluble drug particles in the solvent.

- Tablet coatings- The substances used to coat on the surface of the tablet.

- Disintegrants- The substances used to break the tablet in to small pieces.

- Penetration enhancers- The substances used to facilitate the drug molecules to penetrate from the skin to the blood stream.

- Stabilizing agents - The substances used to increase the stability of the dosage form

- Pharmakon means drug

- Gnosis means knowledge.

- pharmakon, meaning drug,

- poiein meaning make,

- Pharmacopeia meaning any recipe or formula

- **Define Pharmacognosy**:

- De Materia Medica, is considered a milestone in the development of pharmaceutical botany and in the study of naturally occurring medicinal materials.

- This is known as Pharmacognosy now

- **Define Pharmacopeias or formularies**

- Organized sets of monographs and books of these standards are called pharmacopeias or formularies.

- **International Organization for Standardization.-ISO**

It is an International consortium of representative bodies constituted to develop and promote uniform or harmonized international standards.

- **The Mission of Pharmacy**

- The mission of pharmacy is to serve society as the profession responsible for the appropriate use of medications, devices, and services to achieve optimal therapeutic outcomes.

- **Pharmaceutical Care**

- Pharmaceutical care is that component of Pharmacy practice which entails the direct interaction of the pharmacist with the patient for the purpose of caring for that patient's drug-related needs.

Short answer questions

1. What are the qualities of drug?

- Diversity of their actions and effects on the body.

This quality enables their selective use in the treatment of a range of common and rare conditions

2.   Explain about the different sources of drug with examples.

Plant, Animal, Byproducts of microbial growth, or through chemical synthesis, molecular modification or biotechnology.

Plant source: Acetyldigoxin from Digitalis Lanata

☐   Animal source:

☐   Sheep thyroid is a source of thyroxin, used in hypertension.

☐   Byproducts of microbial growth:

☐   Penicillium notatum is a fungus which gives penicillin.

☐   Synthetic Sources:

☐   When the nucleus of the drug from natural source as well as its chemical structure is altered, we call it synthetic.

☐   Examples include Emetine Bismuth Iodide

3. What are four factors necessary for drug discovery?

☐   Computer libraries

☐   and data banks of chemical compounds and

☐   sophisticated methods of screening for potential biologic activity assist drug discovery

☐   Collective contributions of scientific specialists

4. Describe the follow-up processes after discovery of a potential new drug substance.

☐   After a potential new drug substance is discovered and undergoes definitive chemical and physical characterization, a great deal of biologic information must be gathered.

☐   Basic pharmacology,

☐   nature and mechanism of action of the drug on the biologic system,

☐   Toxicological features.

☐   Drug's site and rate of absorption, pattern of distribution and concentration within the body, duration of action, method and rate of its elimination or excretion must be studied.

☐   Drugs metabolic degradation and activity of its metabolites

☐   Short and long term effects of the drug on body cells, tissues and organs

5. What is a difference between drug and poison?

DOSE

6. What do you mean by the term Pharmaceutical ingredients?

☐   In addition to the active therapeutic ingredients, formulation contains non-therapeutic /pharmaceutical ingredients.

7. What are the use of Pharmaceutical ingredients or excipients?

☐   Through their use formulation achieves its unique composition and physical appearance.

6. Mention the NINE factors used to recommend the proper dosage form.

☐   1.stability of a drug in a formulation and its effectiveness through its usual shelf life

☐   2. all components are Physically and chemically compatible,

☐   3. Preserved against decomposition

☐   4. Therapeutic ingredients must be released in proper quantity

☐   5. possess attractive features

☐   6.Properly packaged and clearly labeled

☐   7. Proper administration

☐   8. Reevaluation and adjustments should be made in the dosage, regimen, schedule, form, choice of drug administered.

☐   9. Advise of side effects and of foods, beverages and/or other drugs that may interfere with the effectiveness of the medication

7. What were the two reasons believed by early races causes of diseases?

☐ Early races believed disease was caused by the entrance of demons or evil spirits into the body.

8. What were the treatments followed by early races to cure the diseases?

☐ Treatment was through use of spiritual practices, application of materials and giving herbs or plant materials.

9. How many drugs and formulae were mentioned in the Ebers papyrus?

More than 800 formulas or prescriptions and more than 700 drugs mentioned.

10.What are the botanical substances , minerals and vehicles used by early races?

Botanical substances as acacia, castor bean and fennel are mentioned along with references to minerals like Iron oxide, sodium carbonate, sodium chloride and sulfur.

• Vehicles were beer, wine, milk and honey

11.Match the following:

☐ Hippocrates. -introduction of scientific pharmacy and medicine

☐ Dioscorides, - De Materia Medica,

☐ Galen - perfect system of physiology, pathology and treatment.

☐ Paracelsus. - Botanical science to one based on chemical science.

12. When Pharmacy officially separated from medicine for the first time?

1240 AD

13. What are the required skills for pharmacist?

☐ special knowledge ,

☐   skill,

☐   initiative and

☐   Responsibility if adequate care to the medical needs of the people was to be guaranteed.

14. Define pharmacopeias or formularies

 Organized sets of monographs and books of these standards are called pharmacopeias or formularies

15. The first American Pharmacopeia was the so called Lititz Pharmacopeia, published in 1778.

16. First edition of National Formulary of unofficial preparations was published in 1888

17. All monographs on therapeutically active drug substances appeared in the USP section, whereas all monographs on pharmaceutical agents appeared in the NF section.

18. USP 26 - NF 21 contains approximately 4000 drug monographs.

19. Mention any four parameters given in USP and NF Monographs.

20. In each monograph, the standards set forth are specific to the individual therapeutic agent or dosage form preparation to ensure purity, potency and quality.

21. International Pharmacopeia is published by the World Health Organization of the United Nations.

22. What are the countries have published their own pharmacopeias?

United Kingdom, France, Italy, Japan, India, Mexico, Norway and the former Union of Soviet Socialist Republics

23. Selection of the pharmacopeia by Countries not having a national pharmacopeia is usually based on

geographic proximity,

a common heritage or language, or

a similarity of drugs and pharmaceutical products used

24. ISO standards used in the pharmaceutical industry is ISO-9000-ISO 9004

25. ISO standards used in the institution is ISO-9001-ISO 2000

26. Mention any five roles of a Pharmacist

•   Through professional interaction and communication with other health professionals, the pharmacist can contribute greatly to patient care.

☐   Pharmacist serves the patient as an advisor on drugs and encourages their safe and proper use.

☐   Pharmacist delivers pharmaceutical services in a variety of community and institutional health care

☐   Pharmacist legal responsibility for

procurement,

storage,

control and distribution of effective pharmaceutical products and for the compounding and filling of prescription orders.

Definitions:

1. Granulation

Granulation is the process in which powder particles are made to adhere to form larger particles called granules.

2. Bulk volume

The volume occupied by both powder and air

3. True volume

The volume occupied by only powder

4. Void volume

The volume occupied by air

5. Porosity

The ratio of void volume and bulk volume

6. Bulk density

Mass of powder / bulk volume

7. Nucleation

Further agitation densifies the pendular bodies to form the capillary state and these bodies act as nuclei for further granule growth.

8. Transition

Nuclei can grow by two possible mechanisms:

- Either single particles can be added to the nuclei by pendular bridges or two or more nuclei may combine.

The combined nuclei will be reshaped by the agitation of the bed.

9. Ball growth

Further granule growth produces large, spherical granules

10. Coalescence

- Two or more granules join to form a larger granule.

11. Breakage

Granules break into fragments which adhere to other granules forming a layer of material over the surviving granule

12. Abrasion transfer

- Agitation of the granule bed leads to attrition of material from granules.

This abraded material adheres to other granules, increasing their size

13. Layering

◪ When <u>a second batch of powder mix is added to a bed of granules, the powder will</u> <u>adhere to the granules forming a layer</u> over the surface increasing the granule size.

14. Slugging

◪ After weighing and mixing the ingredients, powder mix. is slugged, or compressed into <u>large flat tablets or pellets about 1'' in dia.</u>

15. Friability

Loss of weight of tablet in container due to removal of fine particles from the surface of the tablet.

16. Hardness

Force required to break the tablet

17) Lubricants

Substance used to reduce the friction between diewall and tablet

18) Glidants

Substance used to reduce the friction between granules

19) Anti-adhesives

Substance used to reduce the friction between tablet / granules and punches.

Short answer questions

1. How can you made the powder to adhere to form granules?

2. What is the relation between the size and number of sieves?

3. What are the two essential properties to be achieved in granulation?

4. What are the parameters used to evaluate flow property and compressibility?

5. Mention the two uses of perfect flow property and one use of compressibility in tablet production.

6. What are the reasons for granulation?

7. Explain about five primary bonding mechanisms.

8. What are reasons for choosing dry granulation method?

9. Draw the flow diagram of dry granulation and wet granulation method.

10. Examples for fillers, disintegrating agents, lubricants and glidants.

11. Which machinery is used to prepare slugs in small scale method?

12. Which machinery is used to prepare slugs as well as ribbon in large scale method?

13. How much pressure is applied in roller compaction?

14. What are the solvents used in wet granulation method?

15. Mention any two disadvantages of using water as solvent in wet granulation method.

16. Mention any two advantages of using water as solvent in wet granulation method.

17. Examples of wet granulators and dry granulators.

PREFORMULATION

Define the following terms:

1.   Spectroscopy

The study of the interaction between matter and radiated energy

2.   Preformulation

Preformulation involves the application of biopharmaceutical principles to the physicochemical parameters of drug substance are characterized with the goal of designing optimum drug delivery system

3.   Biopharmaceutics

The study of physical and chemical properties of drugs and their proper dosage form as related to the onset, duration and intensity of drug action

4.   PKa

Equal amount of lipophilicity and aqueous nature of drug-

Partition coefficient-Penetration & absorption

5.   Polymorph

A polymorph is a solid material with at least two different molecular arrangements each of which gives a distinct crystal species.

6.   Assay

Purity of drug in dosage forms

7.   Solvolysis

The process of reaction between solute and solvent and formation of new compound

8.   Hygroscopicity

Absorption of moisture from air by the drug particles.

9.   Bulk density

Weight of powder/bulk volume

Bulk volume =True volume +void volume

10.   Angle of repose

A static heap of powder, when only gravity acts upon it, will tend to form conical mound. The angle to the horizontal is known as angle of repose.

Answer the following:

1.   Where preformulation studies are done?

2.   What are the Basic Properties to be studied in preformulation phase:

3.   Most drugs absorb light in the ultraviolet wavelengths (190—390 nm) since they are generally aromatic and/or contain double bonds.

4.   Mention four uses of Spectroscopy.

5.   What are the uses of solubility concept in preformulation studies?

6.   What is the use of melting point concept in preformulation studies?

7.   Match the following:

a. Capillary melting – Melting point apparatus

b. Hot stage microscopy - Microscope

c. Differential scanning calorimetric thermal analysis – DSC-Analytical instrument

8.   What are the parameters to be investigated for polymorph in preformulation?

9.   Explain Drug degradation occurs by four main processes.

10.   What are the stress conditions used in preformulation stability assessment studies in solid and aqueous liquid dosage forms?

11.   What are the two major applications of the microscope in pharmaceutical preformulation?

12.   The main goal of preformulation studies is Innovative; stable, safe, cost- effective dosage forms capable of delivering the substance for its intended use.

Definitions:

1. Tablets

▫   Tablets are solid dosage forms usually prepared with the aid of suitable pharmaceutical excipients.

▫   They may vary in size, shape, weight , hardness, thickness, disintegration and dissolution characteristics.

▫   Most tablets are used in the oral administration of drugs.

◻   Many of these are prepared with colorants and coatings of various types.

2.Hardness:

Tablet's tensile strength is measured in terms of load/pressure required to crush it when placed on its edge

3.Thickness:

Depends on the die filling, materials to be compressed by compressional forces.

4.Friability:

Loss in weight of tablets in the containers due to removal of fine particles from their surfaces.

5. Scored tablet

A line or cut on the surface of tablet

6. Antiadherents

Prevent the friction between granules and hopper

7. Glidants

Prevent the friction between punches and granules

8. Lubricants

Prevent the friction between die wall and tablet

9. Loading dose

Immediate release of drug from shell part of multilayered tablet to begin the pharmacological action

10. Maintanence dose

Controlled release of drug from core part of multilayered tablet to sustain the pharmacological action

11. Gelcap

A recent innovation

The innovator product, the gelcap, is a capsule shaped compressed tablet that allows the coated product to be about one-third smaller than a capsule filled with an equivalent amount of powder.

12. Effervescent salts

- Prepared by compressing granular effervescent salts that release gas when in contact with water.

- They generally contain medicinal substances that dissolve rapidly when added to water.

13.Monograms

To mark with a design or one or more letters

14. Lyophilization or freeze drying

Drying under low temperature and high pressure

15. Slugging

After weighing and mixing the ingredients, powder mix. is slugged, or compressed into large flat tablets or pellets about 1'' in dia.

16. Tablet dedusting

To remove traces of loose powder adhering to tablets following compression, tablets are conveyed directly from tableting machine to a deduster.

17. Capping, splitting:

The top or bottom part of the tablet separates from the main body completely or partially.

18. Laminating:

The tablets breaks into two or more horizontal layers.

19. Mottling:

The unequal distribution of colors on the tablet surface.

20. Binding:

Tablets adheres or tear in the die

21. Picking

The materials get off from the tablet surface and adhere to the face of the punches.

22. Sticking

Adherence of granules to die walls

23. Chipping

Breaking of tablet edges

Short answer questions

1. How can you prepare the tablets?

2. What are the advantages and disadvantages of tablets?

3. Explain plate method

4. Give two reasons for the tablets that are not scored.

5. Write about compressed tablets and multi compressed tablets

6. Write the difference between core and shell in multi compressed tablets

7. Mention 4 advantages of sugar coated tablets

8. What are polymers used in film coated tablets?

9. Mention 4 advantages of film coated tablets

10. What are polymers used in enteric coated tablets?

11. Define buccal and sublingual tablets.

12.Write about lozenges.

13. Write the important features of chewable tablets

14. How can you administer the effervescent tablets

15. Write about

    Molded tablets

Tablet triturates

Hypodermic tablets

RDT

Extended release tablets

Vaginal tablets

16. What are the disadvantages of RDT?

<u>Quality Standards and Compendial Requirements</u>

1.How can you perform Tablet weight and USP Weight Variation Test?

2. How can you perform Content Uniformity?

3. Tablet thickness may be measured by <u>hand gauge</u>

4. <u>lozenges and buccal tablets</u>, that are intended to dissolve slowly, intentionally are made <u>hard</u>

5. Other tablets for immediate drug release are <u>made soft.</u>

6. <u>A force of 4 kg</u> is considered minimum requirement for a satisfactory tablet in hardness test.

7. A tablet's durability may be determined through the use of <u>a friabilator</u>

8. How can you perform Friability?

9. Maximum weight loss of not more than <u>1%</u> generally is considered acceptable for most products in friability test.

10. How can you do disintegration test?

11. Define complete disintegration

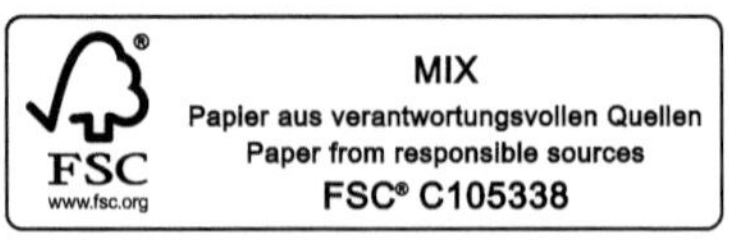

Printed by Books on Demand GmbH, Norderstedt / Germany